Journeys Through Darkness - Extended Edition

An Award-Winning Photographer's Crusade to Find the Light
Through the Darkness of AIDS and Related Blindness

A Biography of AIDS

By Alina Oswald

This book was published by Alina Oswald

SHARED PEN Edition – Second Edition

Photographs by Kurt Weston - Second Edition

Edited by Ira Weitz

Cover Art by Alina Oswald

Cover Photograph, Journey Through Darkness, and other photographs by Kurt Weston

For more information, please visit:

Alina Oswald: www.alina-arts.com

Kurt Weston: www.kurtweston.com

www.SharedPen.com

Also by Alina Oswald:

Infinite Lights: A Collection of 9/11-Related Photography

Vampire Fantasies

Backbone

The Awakening...

The Best of MJ

For Dirk, Mom and Dad

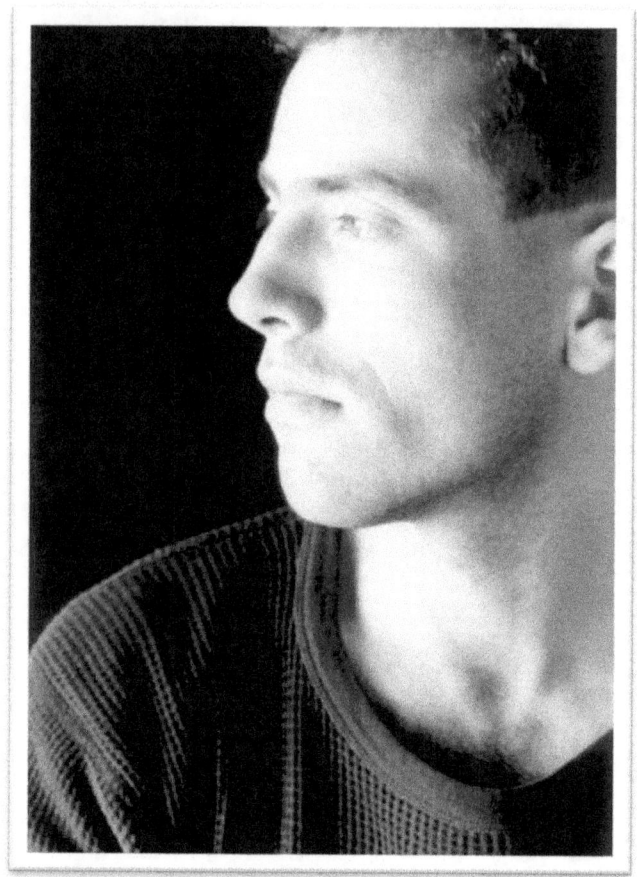

Praise for Journeys Through Darkness

"The story of award-winning photographer, Kurt Weston, who gains his spiritual vision, while losing his physical eyesight, proves that 'life is a mystery to live, not a problem to solve.' To survive and thrive in this world, you have to be tougher than your problem. And it is precisely that toughness which is exhibited by the Warrior and subject of Journeys Through Darkness, Kurt Weston." ~ Ira Weitz, Silly-ologist and creator of the Have-A-Silly children's reggae music CD

"'Don't write about Man,' essayist E. B. White observed, "write about a Man." Alina Oswald does just that in her book, Journeys Through Darkness and does it powerfully, bringing a poet's sensitivity to her prose. Her portrait of Kurt Weston, an award-winning photographer who becomes legally blind from AIDS, brings the reality of the disease home to us." ~ T.J. Banks, author of A Time for Shadows, Catsong (Winner of the 2007 Merial Human-Animal Bond Award), Houdini, and Souleiado

"Alina Oswald gives an enthralling as-told-to account of a vibrant man's struggle living with a debilitating disease and the onset of blindness.[...] Journeys Through Darkness is an inspiration for the AIDS afflicted or for anyone on the threshold of losing color-filled vision." ~ Patricia Spork, Freelance Writer and Digital Photo Artist

"Alina Oswald's biography of Kurt Weston introduces the reader to a subject they may never have encountered before—an artist with AIDS. By striking a balance between writing about the pain of illness and celebrating Kurt's strength, compassion and creation of striking works of art, Journeys Through Darkness helps to reduce the stigma associated with HIV. Kurt's story may serve as a source of inspiration to anyone overcoming challenges in their lives. I am proud that others will have the opportunity to learn, through this biography, about Kurt, an artist whose work is featured in the AIDS Museum's permanent collection. ~ Ashley Grosso, Executive Director, The AIDS Museum

"Journeys Through Darkness is a [...] detailed account of [a photographer's] journey in his life with HIV/AIDS [and related vision loss], an inspiring true story of a man who literally overcame everything. Because of Alina Oswald's descriptiveness, it feels as if the reader is standing beside her book subject, Kurt Weston, throughout each page." ~ Lovari, Singer, Songwriter, Actor

"Journeys is riveting..." Arthur Wooten, author of On Picking Fruit, Fruit Cocktail and Birthday Pie

Foreword: Finding Visionaries

By Guido A. Sanchez, Former Manager and CEO at New York City Metro LGBT and HIV/AIDS Support Organizations

I was once asked why I, someone so young (only a few years past a quarter century), could care so deeply about HIV / AIDS that I would commit my life to it, as the Executive Director of the LGBT Community Center & AIDS Service Organization in Northern New Jersey. The question kind of stumped me, and all I could say was "why not?" How could I, an openly gay and proud man, deny that AIDS is one of the single most important parts of my history, my community's history? AIDS activism continues to suffer today from apathy and puritanism, all the meanwhile our communities are still being decimated, and people are still being infected.

Since AIDS activism rose up within the community-at-large in a very public and graphic way in the mid-1980s, the AIDS community and artists community have had inextricable ties. Artists have tried to represent their experiences with HIV / AIDS (such as the play Angels in America), voice their anger (such as any work by David Wojnarowicz), or force change (such as ACT UP's 'Silence=Death' posters). On a sadder note, there is the undeniable fact that AIDS has decimated our artists community — and anyone who has been a part of the movement has to ask themselves, how many future leaders, painters, writers, singers, dancers, creators, mentors, etc. have we lost to the virus over the last twenty-five plus years?

Not all of these visionaries were lost, and photographer Kurt Weston has chosen to share his own journey through darkness in his life and work, with the help of biographer Alina Oswald. I first met Alina when she came to our Community Center to write one of her many articles on HIV / AIDS activism and the social service landscape. Alina's dedication to the grassroots work around HIV has brought her to offer her services as a photographer, and luckily even display some of her art photography in a show at our gallery. This book brings together so many pieces of her vision for a world without AIDS. I've never had the opportunity to meet Kurt, but now I feel like I understand artist's vision much more. Kurt's openness about his status and his experience, and the way he synergizes that into his art, is a moving inspiration. Kurt cites in the book that he is inspired by those who are inspired by reason, intellect, and compassion, and as Alina weaves his story for us, we see those three traits, and so much more, as Kurt navigates his life as an artist living with HIV. Alina takes us on a journey with Kurt, as we find his artistic vision grow stronger when his vision becomes impaired through AIDS medication, and as his life takes unexpected and surprising turns, all of which he navigates with grace, integrity, and above all, passion.

Now when I get asked how I can devote so much of my energy to AIDS activism, I know I can say that Kurt is the reason I do what I do. Kurt's ability to inspire, and then to humbly cite his own source of inspiration as others who glean their own inspiration from reason and compassion. That someone's ability to journey through darkness, and to maintain an immovable passion for helping others journey through that same darkness, to help people travel beyond their fears, hatred, prejudices, and find that light, could be woven into an inspiring tale, that is why we need people like Kurt and Alina. That is why we need stories like this. Now instead of saying, "why not fight with every breath I take" I know what I can say instead.

Guido A. Sanchez, 2008

Table of Contents

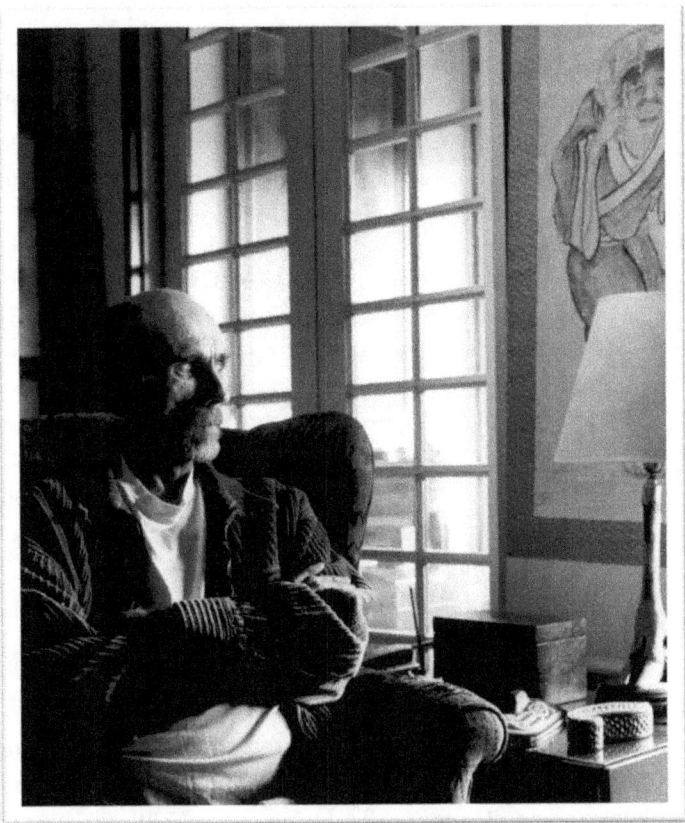

Introduction

The photograph featured an old man sitting in a chair, with his back at a tall glass door. The weak daylight poured inside the room to mingle with the pale artificial light of a night lamp. Wide and white, glowing within the shadows, the man's eyes became yet another source of light in the photograph. With his face drawn and his eyes haunted, he seemed unaware of the mist of shadow and light surrounding him. Rather he gazed beyond the visual sphere of the photograph, as if he found himself at the crossroads between two realms, about to follow a path unfolding in front of him, into some mysterious unknown.

The man in the photograph—his eyes, in particular— haunted me for weeks and months to follow. His story was a mystery to me. At the time there was no way for me to know that I was to embark on a journey of discovery, a journey that would help me unveil his mystery.

I browsed through the Unfinished Works website where the award winning photograph was posted. A few clicks brought me to the story of The Last Light, an image that, as I found out, was the artwork of a visual artist called Kurt Weston.

It so happened that, at the time, I was looking for an artist to interview for an AIDS-related publication. I had found the Unfinished Works website several months earlier and bookmarked it specifically for its Last Light, which now seemed to light the path to the possible subject of my article. Therefore, I emailed Kurt Weston and, luckily for me, he agreed to give me the interview.

Months later I had the opportunity to travel to the West Coast to take part in a celebration of life and triumph over AIDS, as a guest at Joel Rothschild's party. Diagnosed with AIDS on April 22nd, 1986, Rothschild—an AIDS activist, long-term survivor and bestselling author—believes in the power of living in the moment. He talks about that in his books, Signals—A Story of Life After Life and Hope—A Story of Triumph.

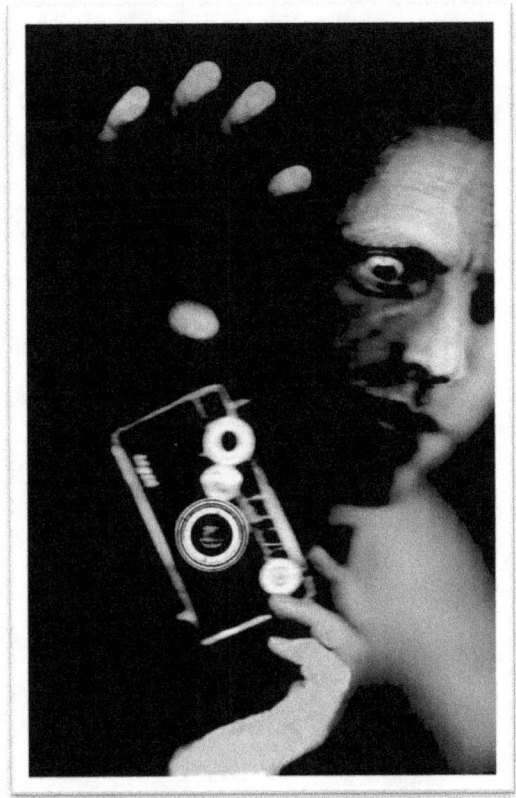

Eye of the Beholder

While on the West Coast, I also had the chance to meet Kurt Weston and his partner, Terry Roberts. What followed was an immersion into the visual artist's world, as I followed Kurt Weston's journey into darkness and his struggle to rediscover the light.

Alina Oswald, 2010

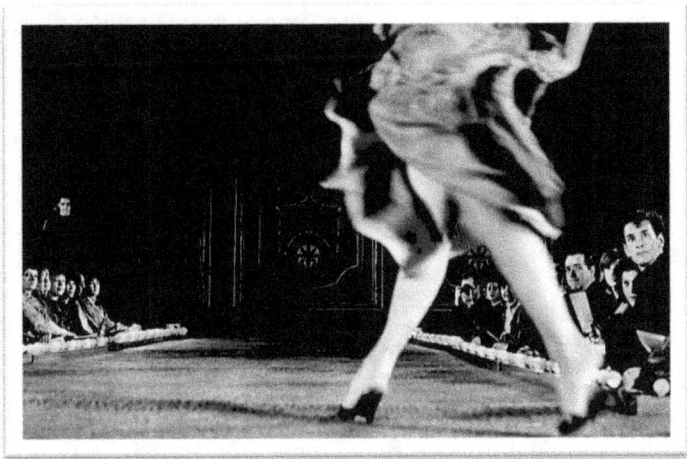

Chapter One: The Runway

*Preview of a Plague: Glitz, Glamour and Glory of Fashion
Photography*

"All aboard!"

I've always thought of these two words as being part
of some script, a symbol of departure, separation, tears and
heartache... an ending. I've never thought of them as actually
being used in real life. But there I was, on an early summer
morning, in my own reality, the first time on a train in over
fifteen years, settled comfortably in my seat.

"All aboard!"

The two magic words set the train in motion, the
conductor's voice still ringing in my ears as the train pulled

slowly out of New York City's Penn Station, heading to D.C. But, unlike the movies, my first Amtrak experience was not the farewell-y, teary kind, but quite the opposite. In a peculiar way, it symbolized the beginning of a journey and the start of a spiritual transformation.

I was on my way to attend the VSA Arts gallery opening event, personally invited by Kurt Weston. He was one of the twenty-three featured artists selected from a group of 560 artists from around the world.

Formally known as Very Special Arts and founded in 1974 by Ambassador Jean Kennedy Smith, VSA Arts is an international nonprofit organization promoting and showcasing the works of artists with disabilities from over sixty countries. Kurt Weston is not only a VSA Arts featured artist but also a member of VSA's Board of Directors in California. Each year he attends the annual VSA National Convention in Washington, D.C.

As part of the event Kurt Weston and his partner, gay rights and AIDS activist Terry Roberts, attended in 2005, there was also an art show displaying works created by children with disabilities. One of the winners was a girl from California who, while paralyzed from the neck down, could paint by holding the brush in her mouth.

At this event it is not unusual for Kurt and Terry to meet with senators and to advocate for the continuation of funding for the arts and education, funding which is vital for the careers of many potentially good artists. It was during a reception following one of these meetings that the visual artist had the chance to meet Senator Ted Kennedy, his sister Jean Kennedy Smith and Senator John Kerry.

The three were squeezing their way through the reception room as everyone present reached out to shake their hands and greet them. As Kurt Weston took his turn to shake Ted Kennedy's hand, the director of VSA Arts California, who was also present at the reception, took a snapshot of the quick handshake for which, even today, Weston considers himself lucky.

When he first mentioned the 2006 VSA Arts event to me, I was hesitant. I guess because it wasn't something that happened to me everyday. Kurt Weston's artwork has fascinated me ever since I first set my eyes on The Last Light, even if only through the samples posted on the artist's website. But I had never had the opportunity to look at the actual photographs and touch them, and try to connect with them. The VSA Arts event opening provided me with this very unique opportunity, and there was no way I was going to miss it.

And so, on a glorious weekend in early June 2006, I found myself for the first time on the Amtrak. The train trip itself ended up being a surprisingly positive experience; the weekend, an artistic adventure.

One of Weston's winning entries welcomed us— Kurt, Terry and myself—as we first entered the Kennedy Center for the Performing Arts, where the event took place. The featured photograph, Losing the Light, is part of Weston's Blind Vision series of self-portraits capturing the artist's vision of his blindness, showing people the physical and emotional impact that visual loss can have on an individual.

AIDS-related retinitis has left the photographer totally blind in his left eye and only with some limited peripheral vision in his right eye. Therefore, he cannot focus or see things clearly anymore. He can only make out tones of colors. He also experiences floaters, or what he describes as "pieces of cotton that are stuck in my eye and keep floating and flashing every time I move my eye."

While searching for a way to represent this visual disturbance, Kurt Weston decided to use something obstructive in the photograph to block the viewers from seeing his face in the image. The result was a series of self-portraits known today as the Blind Vision series. He ended up taking each photograph in this series sitting behind a glass sprayed with foaming glass cleaner. He started by spraying the foam all over the glass, and then he wiped the foam away with his hand or sometimes just let it drip. He then pressed his face and hands against the glass, while taking the photographs through the glass, using a camera with a self-timer. "You see my hand pushing away the foam, which is what I would love to do," he says explaining the technique. "I would like to be able to wipe away all that cotton that keeps floating in front of my eye and get a clear view of what I want to see out in the world."

On that early summer evening, the sunset light poured through the tall windows of the Kennedy Center of Performing Arts building, glowing onto Kurt Weston's Losing the Light and bringing me even closer to the photograph. I could see the artist's face and fingertips pressing against glass trying to push away the foam, but I couldn't recognize him. I reached out and aligned my fingertips with the foamy imprints. And they almost overlapped, briefly pulling me inside the photograph, allowing me to see the world through the artist's eyes, from within its blackness.

Unfortunately, I couldn't hang around for too long because there were too many people around me, pulling me out of my reverie. Besides, we had to move farther to other images, sculptures and paintings in the gallery.

Soon, I found more of Weston's works. They were two digital images, part of a more recent body of work, which the artist calls the Visual Assist series. One of the images in this series shows the photographer holding an old camera. I wondered if it was the same camera he was cradling in his hand as he walked next to Terry and me. He would snap pictures, talk to people, admire others' works and sign cards for those lined up to get his autograph. At times he would hand the camera to his partner and pose for pictures with members of VSA Arts and other artists.

Kurt and Terry have been together for many years. They belong together. Their relationship is a bridge, a connection some call "oneness" that can survive the physical existence and continue into the vast beyond that follows.

Someone once said that people who live together for a long time and who belong together start looking alike... Maybe it's true. I recognized these subtle "similarities" in

Terry, who was wearing a navy blue suit with tie to match, and also in Kurt, dressed up in black slacks and shirt and a gray jacket.

The two men are approximately the same age, same height at about six feet two, with their hair trimmed almost military style. They move flawlessly together and finish each other's sentences.

Maybe the best term to describe the couple would be "gentleness." While Kurt is the communicator, Terry is the quiet, almost shy, kind of person ready to escape the large crowds in order to focus on more important things, like making everybody feel at home even in the strangest of places. He'd be the one offering someone his chair or bringing somebody a cup of coffee or something to eat from the snack table and he would not rest until making sure everybody is set and content.

As we walked around the gallery and admired the works of artists from the United States, South Africa, Australia and other places, Kurt started to snap pictures left and right. And watching his hands cradle the camera with much care, I wondered how many of the images would end up in his portfolio. After all, it was with that dark and aged Nikon that Weston started his career in photography and, with it, the beginning of his journey to become the innovative visual artist he is today.

***

Kurt Weston bought the Nikon camera in 1983, when he was preparing to go back to school, to pursue his second degree—a Bachelor's of Fine Arts in photography from Chicago's Columbia College. At the time, he was working in fashion merchandising and attending various fashion shows was part of his job. At one of these events, he brought his (then) brand new camera along with him and snapped a few pictures. One of the images, The Runway, is now part of his visual art portfolio and it marks the beginning of his career in photography.

Weston's passion for photography started early in life, when his high school offered, for the very first time, a photography course which utilized a darkroom with a full complement of essential equipment. That marked his first contact with the world of real photography. Years later, while in college and still debating on what his major was going to be, an art history course reintroduced Weston to photography and, thus, jumpstarted his interest in an artistic pursuit. But following that dream was no easy matter.

"How the hell are you gonna make a living being an artist?" his father asked when Kurt first expressed his interest in pursuing a career in the arts. So, because his father was paying for his education at the time (1975), Kurt decided to enroll in Fashion Merchandising at Northern Illinois University, in the town of DeKalb, Illinois. It sounded like a great idea, because to work in the fashion merchandising industry, Kurt could mix the artistic creativity he loved, to determine what was "in fashion," with the sense of business he needed to develop in order to determine how best to sell fashion merchandises and, therefore, to make money and achieve the stability his father was talking about.

Weston graduated from Northern Illinois University in 1979 and landed a marketing job in the staff service division at Hart Schaffner and Marx, a famous brand clothing and suit manufacturing company in Chicago with a century-old tradition, known today as Hartmarx. But the excitement of taking the first steps towards a safe and stable career path in fashion merchandizing was short lived. Two years into his first job, Weston started to become increasingly disappointed with his work and realized he was ready for something more exciting. So he quit Hart Schaffner and Marx and started looking for something else.

His second job was also in the fashion industry, but this time in retail. Weston ended up managing a custom shirt shop. And yet again, it didn't take long for his second job to become less enlightening and less interesting than he had hoped it would be.

The experience brought him even more disappointment with his profession and with his career choice. Suddenly, the safety net his professional path was offering him slipped into second place, while his desire to do something he really loved took priority. Kurt realized that, despite his experience with his two jobs in fashion merchandising, his passion for the arts, in particular for photography, had remained intact. And because by then, his father's obligation to finance his education was through—as a matter of fact, by then his father was pretty much out of

Kurt's life—the future photographer decided to follow his heart and the artistic pursuit he'd always desired.

So, in 1983 Weston quit his job at the custom shirt shop, took out school loans and enrolled in a Bachelor's in Fine Arts degree at Chicago's Columbia College to study photography. He went to school full-time and devoted all his time and energy to his studies. And he excelled in all of his courses. Nowadays, the artist attributes his excellent grades to the exuberant sense of liberation and enthusiasm he felt as he began studying what he really loved.

Kurt graduated from Columbia College in 1985 and took a job as an assistant to a commercial photographer for Stephens Biondi and Decicco—the studio is no longer in business, but in its day it was one of the largest and most famous product photography studios in the Chicago area. At Stephens Biondi and Decicco, Kurt ended up working with a senior photographer—his first "mentor"—who had some forty years experience in the industry and an eye for new talent, and who saw a promising future in Kurt's work.

While in school, Kurt had studied, in particular, art photography. It was something he was interested in, but the established visual artists were not many. Meanwhile, although commercial photography was not art photography, it helped pay Kurt's bills faster and easier. So, while he was still paying off his student loans, he had to stick to his job. And doing so, he learned a lot about lighting, in particular the special lighting necessary for food photography, also about building a room design and other similar things. In time, he got to work on various projects for companies like G.E., Siemens, for television and food companies.

For a while, he found his first job as a commercial product photographer extremely interesting, offering him the opportunity to learn as much about photography as he could... which he did. But two years into his work, Weston started, yet again, to become frustrated with his work and bored with the monotonous subject matter of commercial product photography.

Around that time he happened to bump into a friend, a former colleague from Columbia College. They chatted for a while and caught up with their lives and professions. That's how Kurt learned that his friend was working as a darkroom photographer for a company called Pivot Point International—an international fashion photography company with innovative ideas and with decades of tradition working with successful designers who create in the realm of hair design, esthetics, and nails.

When inquiring about possible job openings, Kurt found out that Pivot Point was actually looking for a second person to work in the darkroom. And although it wasn't much of a step forward in his career as a photographer, he considered the possible job an opportunity and applied for it.

Shortly afterwards he got hired as a darkroom photographer. He was to make fashion photography prints. Soon, his experience in the fashion industry and his degree in fashion merchandising were to prove helpful in his new job.

While at Pivot Point, Kurt Weston met and got to know many famous industry people like hair stylists, fashion designers and makeup artists. As he was interested to learn more about fashion photography, Weston asked them if it was possible to do a few weekend photography sessions with the models. He volunteered as their weekend photographer. In exchange, he could use the images for his portfolio, as could the models for their own portfolios. The hair stylists and the other industry people and models liked the idea.

One of the company's trademarks has always been an industry-specific book called Design Forum. To this day, Pivot Point International produces three issues of Design Forum every year. Each book includes information on the latest trends in hairstyling techniques, introduces new talents from the industry's finest hair designers and offers students practical tips. Design Forum books are also brimming with professional photographs of cutting-edge, international hair fashion trends.

While Kurt Weston was working in the darkroom and doing the free weekend photography shoots, Pivot Point was working on one of their Design Forum issues and it just happened that they ran out of pictures for that particular book. They also realized that the photos they originally wanted to include in the book weren't really what they were looking for. To add to their problem, the model they wanted to use was nowhere to be found. Neither was the Pivot Point fashion photographer who'd taken the original pictures. Meanwhile, the deadline was approaching and the book was yet to be finished and they were running out of options.

...Or so they thought until the hairstylist who worked with Kurt during the weekends mentioned their freelance photo shoots and showed them a few samples with the model Pivot Point was looking for, wearing a hairstyle he thought would work great for the book. The Design Forum producers took a peek at the pictures and were amazed how much better the hair, and also the photography, looked. Therefore they decided to use Kurt's images in order to complete the project on time. That issue of Design Forum was, as always, a success.

Kurt Weston became their full-time fashion photographer. He was finally making enough money as a photographer to create the stability his father had been talking about. He was finally able to pay off his student loans, buy a three-bedroom condominium in Chicago and do something he loved with his profession.

At Pivot Point he had his own studio and his own team of hairstylists, fashion designers and makeup artists. He was in charge of making everybody feel comfortable and at ease during the photo shoots and he was getting along wonderfully with the people he worked with. And he was definitely getting along with his job. He was enthusiastic and excelled in his photography. He also traveled to many fashion shows across the U.S. and Europe and he got to work with brand names like Clairol, Matrix, Helene Curtis and the like.

Kurt Weston worked for Pivot Point International for a few years, from the late eighties to the early nineties. While his career as a fashion photographer was soaring, many of his friends were losing their battle with a mysterious virus that was threatening—and, ultimately, claiming—their lives. There was no cure and nobody, not even the medical experts, knew what was really causing the increasing numbers of sick and dying young men.

While the photographer didn't have any symptoms of the disease, he had many reasons to suspect that he, too, could be infected. Yet, he wasn't eager to find out if he had the virus because there was no cure in sight. The only treatment available was AZT, which had too many powerful side effects. Medical professionals had much to learn about the virus and what they knew at the time wasn't really enough to ease the patients' suffering… or to save their lives. Therefore, knowing one's HIV status usually meant living the short time one had left in suffering, pain, and depression. And Weston refused to do that.

By 1991 the number of AIDS-related deaths skyrocketed. Many of Kurt's friends and people he knew in his community became infected with HIV. But Kurt didn't really worry. He had been feeling fine and hadn't been sick at all, so there hadn't been any reason for him to go to the doctor for his annual physical. As a matter of fact, Kurt hadn't been to a doctor in over a decade. He'd been healthy… at least up until the end of October 1991, when he started coughing. It was a persistent cough, exhausting, draining him of energy.

Not knowing what to make of it, Kurt tried to self-diagnose, thinking he had an allergy. So, he decided to put to good use the health insurance he had through his work and flipped through the provider books with their endless lists of physicians, searching for an allergist. He found one and called his office to make an appointment. A few days later the doctor gave Kurt several shots of different allergens under his skin to determine just what he was allergic to, and then sent him home, advising him to return in a few days.

Once at home, Kurt started feeling much worse. He went to bed only to wake up in the middle of the night soaked in his own sweat. That's when he realized that something was seriously wrong with him and it wasn't allergies. He started to think that whatever was wrong had something to do with HIV.

Only a week earlier Kurt had taken his date to a gay bar, where he first noticed an AIDS magazine. He picked it up and flipped through its pages and he came upon a list of various opportunistic infections associated with AIDS. One of them was Pneumocystis carinii pneumonia, or PCP, otherwise known as "the AIDS pneumonia." Kurt mentioned his suspicion regarding his HIV status, but the other guy brushed him away, saying that Kurt was probably overreacting.

But after waking up several nights covered in sweat and feeling sicker and weaker by the minute, Kurt decided to call a doctor—a general practitioner this time—and make an appointment. He got in a few days later and by then he was coughing constantly and had mild fever.

The doctor x-rayed Kurt's lungs and drew blood to send out for fast testing. It turned out that the photographer had pneumonia, but the doctor needed more time to determine what kind of pneumonia it was.

Kurt's blood test results were back in no time. The physician studied them and noticed that his patient's white cell count was way out of the normal range. That was reason enough to ask permission to perform an HIV test. Permission granted, the doctor drew more blood from Kurt's arm and sent it out for more testing, and then he sent his patient home with a prescription for antibiotics to treat his pneumonia. Kurt was to return in a week for a follow-up visit.

During the following days, despite the doctor's treatment, he started feeling even worse and by the end of the week Kurt became certain of his HIV status. When it was time for him to return to the doctor's office, his sister insisted on going with him. "You can't go in there without some emotional support," she said and drove him and stood by his side as he received the news.

According to the new blood test results, Kurt not only had HIV. He had AIDS. He was also experiencing his first bout of PCP—two more were to follow in less than a year. His T cell count was fifteen. [In comparison, the T cell count for a healthy person is approximately one thousand or more, measured per unit of blood.]

Being a general practitioner, the physician thought it was time to turn his patient to an HIV specialist, and so he sent Kurt immediately to the hospital. There, although doctors didn't tell Kurt much else at the time, they told the photographer's mother that her son might not make it through the night.

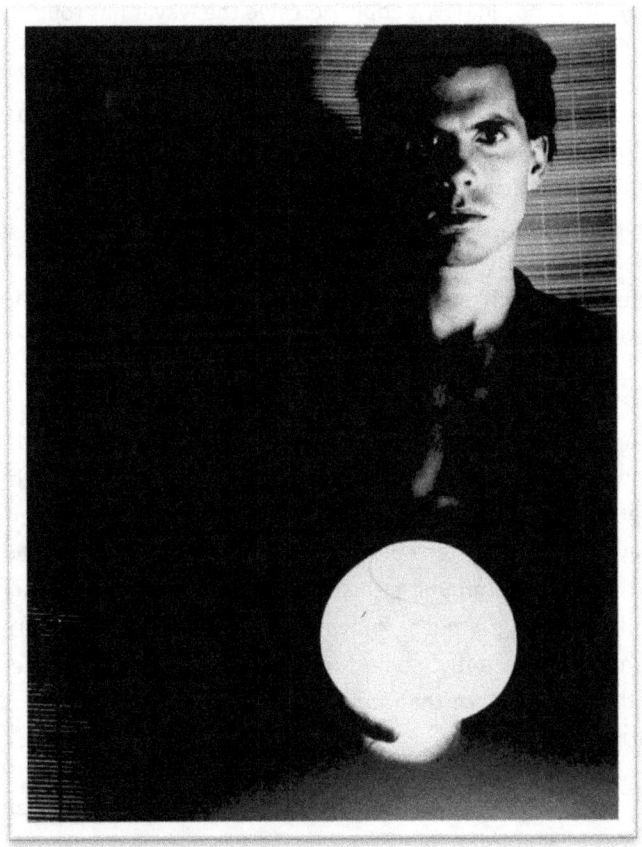

Chapter Two: Cold Warning

The Apparition of a Plague: One Killer Virus, One World

"I'm not clocked down on AIDS," Kurt Weston says talking about the age of AIDS. The pandemic made headlines in the eighties, but it may be much older. Yet, does it make any difference in how people perceive the way it has touched millions of lives?

It may be hard sometimes to realize that it all started with one genetic transformation from a monkey virus to a human one, from one chimpanzee to one human, possibly a monkey hunter in the jungles of Central Africa sometime in the late 1930s. That one mutation has led to the first HIV infection, which medical professionals officially recorded in 1959.

The infected hunter, the world's AIDS patient zero, left his village for the large cities of Africa and the opportunities they provided. The crowds and busy city nightlife attracted both the hunter and his virus in different ways. Soon, HIV started to spread from person to person, taking over communities, cities, countries and continents, and becoming what's known today as the global AIDS pandemic. Presently, some forty million people are infected with HIV and more than twenty million have already died of AIDS, worldwide.

The first U.S. casualties surfaced in June 1981, in Los Angeles, where doctors found a strange type of pneumonia, called Pneumocystis carinii pneumonia in five young gay men. PCP is a type of pneumonia caused by a microorganism that occurs naturally in the lungs of people and animals. Although the medical professionals didn't know the cause of the disease, they knew it was associated with a weakened immune system. And the cause for this impaired immunity was still a mystery. The patients died within days.

That same summer, an article published in the New York Times announced the appearance of a rapidly fatal form of a rare cancer that doctors had found in forty-one homosexual men. A CBS newscaster also reported that a strange cancer seemed to be spreading in the gay community and that nobody knew where it came from or how it was spread.

It was only a blip in the news, but Kurt Weston heard it as he was watching TV in his condo in Chicago. The photographer wondered if he could actually get the strange "gay cancer" and he called his friend, David, who was living in the same neighborhood. His friend had no idea about the mysterious disease threatening their community, but he agreed with Kurt that the gay cancer news was indeed scary news.

It wasn't until a few years later that the "gay cancer" made headlines again, under a new name. In 1985 the Center of Disease Control announced that it wasn't a (gay) cancer causing all the disease and suffering and death, but a virus called Human Immunodeficiency Virus, or HIV. The CDC called the multitude of strange diseases the virus caused Acquired Immune Deficiency Syndrome, or AIDS.

In the late eighties, after David's lover died of AIDS-related causes, Kurt reminded his friend of the CBS report from back in 1981:

"David, do you think you have AIDS?" Kurt asked.

"I think we all have AIDS," David answered.

He died the following year. He was Kurt's first close friend to die of AIDS.

The early eighties were the years of silent sufferings and mysterious deaths. They were the years when a lot of people just... disappeared. One day they were around, the next they were just gone, and nobody knew for sure what had happened to them. It took four years of too many silent deaths and one publicized celebrity death for AIDS to make the headlines in the U.S. It wasn't until the disease claimed the life of a movie star, Rock Hudson, that the threat of the virus was brought home to many Americans.

But that doesn't mean that the first four years of loss and suffering and sickness of unknown people were forgotten. The early eighties have inspired many artists to capture the epidemic in various forms of art, from literature and Broadway shows to film and photography.

Those living in New York City at the time may remember the giant billboard posted in Times Square displaying a picture of Ronald Reagan, his face covered with purple Kaposi's sarcoma lesions. It was a protest message capturing the Reagan Administration's response to the AIDS issue. A quarter century into the pandemic, the picture was reprinted on the cover of POZ magazine.

Kurt Weston lived through the early days of the AIDS epidemic, when people were getting infected and having to deal with the reality that they were sick, victims of the mysterious "gay cancer" and that there was nothing that they could do to stay alive. He had to watch helplessly how his friends were dying horrible and silent deaths, a lot of times having no idea what exactly was killing them, or how, or why. In only a few years AIDS has claimed the lives of everybody the photographer knew in Chicago. And when it didn't claim lives, AIDS isolated and stigmatized its victims.

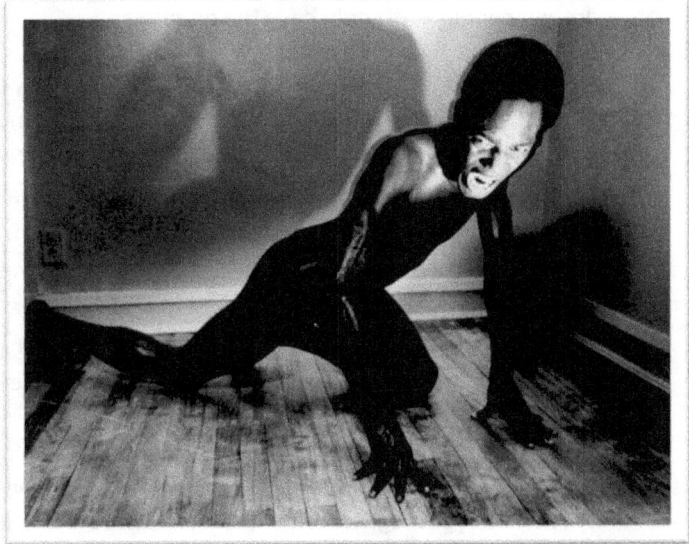

Anger is an Energy

While many of those infected were too weak and sick to leave their beds, others were struggling to maintain some connection to the world outside their homes and their disease. Young men looking three times their age walked the streets, their faces drawn and covered with purple blotches, their emaciated bodies hunched over their canes. They were the messengers of the strange and scary disease, and living proof of its presence in the American society.

But nobody wanted to be around the disease or anybody carrying it. So, many started avoiding using public restrooms or drinking from water fountains, afraid to touch or be around people who could have the disease.

Kurt Weston still recalls the tragedy of those days, the related stigma and harassment, the hysteria, the fear and panic, and also the various personality trends that AIDS brought out in people. A few years after the disease was officially named, one of Kurt's friends stopped by an ATM machine and started to cough while working on his transaction. Someone passing by identified him as being gay and, hearing him cough, called him a "faggot," shouting "Because of you, faggots, we cannot have normal sex anymore."

Today, the events of the early eighties seem like an eternity ago to the photographer. He describes that particular period of time as a pretty wild one, when, despite the "gay cancer" news, people were still maintaining their active lifestyles going out to clubs and having numerous one-night stands. Why wouldn't they? After all, nobody knew the real cause of the gay cancer. By then nobody knew that it was actually a virus causing all the illness and the debilitating death.

When the gay cancer news was first announced, many were not interested in long-lasting, meaningful relationships, but rather in casual encounters. HIV came to the States not long after the gay revolution of the late seventies. And the early eighties found many members of the gay community still celebrating their recently won freedom as they were trying to explore their newfound liberties.

"A lot of times you'd meet someone and then never see him again," Weston explains. "It was kinda like casual contact that would never really turn into much more. That kinda stuff, for me, doesn't exist anymore. I have no desire to go back to that kind of living. But during the eighties it was a lot easier for a person to come and go into your life and not really have any major connection to him."

And, indeed, Weston had few close friends, but that didn't mean that he didn't know lots of people. And he learned that many of those he had casual contact with were getting really sick and dying. It wasn't until later in his life that the photographer started to make deeper, more meaningful relationships with people he got to know through the AIDS community he became part of, while attending AIDS organizations. He became a volunteer at Chicago's Test Positive Aware where, in 1993, he founded Surviving With AIDS Network, or SWAN, an AIDS support group.

But the beginning of the AIDS epidemic did not instantly mark the foundation of an AIDS community in America, especially not outside the epicenters of the epidemic, in cities like Los Angeles, San Francisco and New York City. Gay people gathered together to find a common voice as a community only later, when organizations like ACT-UP (founded in New York City in 1987) started to come along and when its members took their anger and energy to the streets in response to the government's indifference towards the AIDS problem.

This kind of street anger fueled Kurt's inspiration, which, through his camera lenses, became positive energy, which in turn gave him hope and strength to survive the epidemic. Kurt Weston's Anger is an Energy is only one example of the artist's body of work inspired by the events of that time—the administration's lack of response to the epidemic, the "conspiracy theory" fueled by the unbearable effects that AIDS medications had on the African American community and both on Weston's partner and friends receiving a frequently fatal HIV diagnosis.

Most of the time, HIV infected people just wanted to hide from society because they knew they were carrying in their bodies a virus that was giving them an awful disease that was leading to a slow and agonizing death. The feelings of hopelessness and fear manifested exponentially and more intensely during the beginning of the epidemic, when almost nothing was known about the virus. As a result, many people who were not infected or who did not consider themselves part of the "at risk groups" acted out on that fear, prejudice and stigma that surround the subject of HIV/AIDS to this day.

A sick gay person wasn't exactly welcome in his own community either, because gay people were also afraid. Nobody wanted the disease, the virus or anybody it infected. Being gay and infected didn't open any doors or win immediate acceptance in the community. Like mostly everybody else, many gay people didn't want to be around other gay people who had AIDS. Mostly everybody was interested in having a good time, lots of fun partying and being with the beautiful ones. Nobody wanted to be around the sick and dying, or with those whose faces and bodies had been mutilated by the virus, deformed and disfigured by the disease.

"So, most of the people who got infected during the eighties just kinda went away and died," Weston says, "because they didn't want anybody to see them that way." It wasn't until a lot of people started being sick before the gay community decided to do something about the situation, because it was getting alarming.

Kurt's relationship with his friend, Darryl, brought out in the photographer the feeling of fear and avoidance many others felt when it came to HIV/AIDS. It also marked Kurt's first close encounter with the disease itself.

It was right around the time when the CDC officially announced the discovery of the virus that causes AIDS. By then gay people in particular were very well aware that something terrible was happening in their community, because too many of them were starting to die or disappear.

At the time, Kurt Weston was still in Chicago, studying photography at Columbia College. He also had a friend, Darryl, who was a really hot, gorgeous and great-in-bed kinda guy. Kurt and Darryl used to hang around together, spending lots of fun time in bed and nightclubs. Then, one day, without any notice, Darryl was gone. He seemed to have disappeared from Kurt's life.

It wasn't until a year later that Darryl called again, out of the blue, taking Kurt completely by surprise... a nice surprise, the photographer admits. So when Darryl mentioned that he'd like to see him again, Kurt was more than delighted and also excited to the possibilities coming his way. He even offered to photograph his former lover and already started planning and preparing the photo shoot.

But when Darryl showed up at his door, Kurt's excitement turned into horror. The movie star looks were gone, exposing a skeleton-thin Darryl, with his muscles wasted and his skin blotchy. His face was drawn and his fabulous looks vanished.

The sight of his friend left Kurt speechless. He found himself staring helplessly and horrified at an unrecognizable Darryl, wondering what had happened to him. He kept wondering if something was seriously wrong with his friend. And the more Kurt stared, the more certain he became that he didn't want to have anything to do with the man standing in his apartment. "I don't know if he realized how much he'd changed because he didn't act like he was aware that he didn't look physically the way he looked when I first met him," the photographer recalls.

Because he had already promised to do it, Kurt went on with the photo shoot. He did it quickly, despite the fact that he had, first, to change the entire setting in order to shadow the lesions on Darryl's face. And once he was done,

Kurt was glad to see Darryl gone. Only much later he realized that Darryl might have had AIDS when he last saw him, yet he would never really know for sure.

Kurt Weston's second contact with the disease was a much personal and scarier one. It happened in 1985 when his partner at the time found out he was infected.

Kurt had met John entirely by chance, through his friend, David, who was living in the same neighborhood. One day, David called Kurt to tell him that he was coming over. Only he didn't show up alone. On his way to Kurt's place, he stopped by a shopping mall where he bumped into an old friend of his, who was accompanied by a buddy, called John. So the three of them stopped by Kurt's place and later, when it was time to leave, John made sure to exchange phone numbers with Kurt.

John was an up and coming performing artist. He was a talented singer on his way to becoming a big name in the Chicago area. Finding out he was infected changed his career path and the course of his entire life. In 1985 there was nothing to treat the disease, so those infected knew they would probably die. The HIV diagnosis sent him into a deep depression, which incapacitated his professional life for many long years.

When Kurt found out that John was HIV positive, he assumed that he was also infected. In the days and months to follow, the photographer could only witness his own future, as it appeared in his partner's life with the disease and in the way the virus was devastating every aspect of his existence.

Because Kurt didn't want to follow in his partner's footsteps, he never really wanted to find out for sure his own HIV status. Knowing it could bring only agony and the prospect of a near and horrifying death.

John's HIV news came into Kurt's life like a chilling apparition, which the photographer later captured in a portrait of his partner. He called the image Cold Warning. "Imagine someone coming into your room when you're asleep, and taking you by surprise," Kurt Weston explains the photograph and, thus, his feelings relative to the news of his partner's HIV status.

Like many of Weston's photographs, Cold Warning uses shades of light and darkness. The only light source in the photograph comes up from the side to intensify the chilling occurrence of the disease as was the virus news itself reflected on John's face and, thus, in Kurt's life.

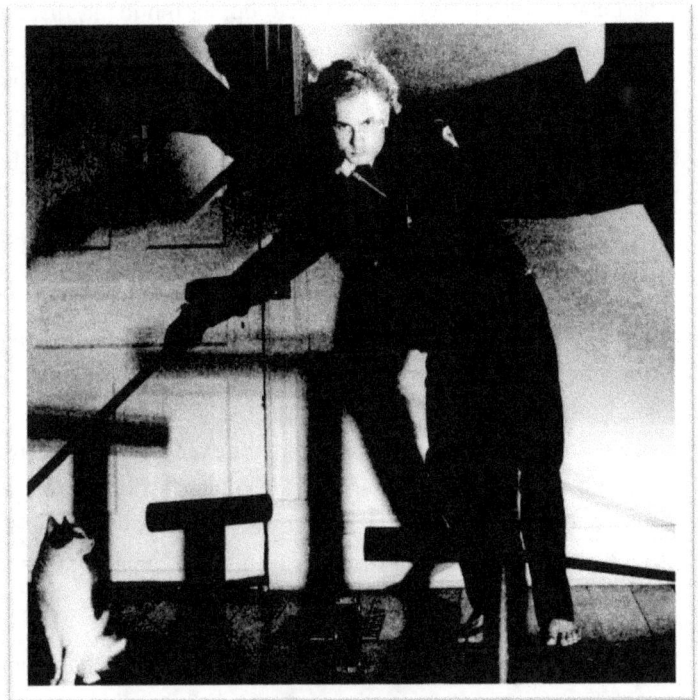

Chapter Three: Dark Angel

The Messenger of Death Is Here: Light, Darkness… and an Accidental Cat

"Maybe there's strength in denial," Kurt Weston says, explaining his mother's inability to accept his "death sentence" diagnosis back in 1991. A Lithuanian immigrant, his mother experienced the Second World War, TB and hepatitis as she was trying to get out of a war-torn Europe and leave behind her homeland, which was to become forever associated with people being blown up, with hunger, disease and other war atrocities. She came to the States as a displaced person, forced to start her life over again in a safe, yet unfamiliar land of opportunities and promises. She had to learn a new language and new ways of living in order to be able to integrate in the American society. And she succeeded, partly because of her survival abilities, which she believes are forever imprinted in her genes.

So in late November 1991, when Kurt's doctor told her that the oldest of her three children might not survive his fatal disease, she refused to accept the grim prognosis. She could not accept defeat and she did not expect her son to just give up when faced with any of the obstacles fate threw at him, even when they were spelled H-I-V, and A-I-D-S, and D-e-a-t-h. She had survived them all—disease, pain, loss—and she knew that Kurt could do it, too.

Sitting by his hospital bed, she grabbed his hand and said, "You're my son and you're strong. You got this strength from my genes and you're not going to die, because you, too, are a survivor."

But in that particular moment, the photographer didn't feel anything like a survivor. He didn't know what his future was going to bring him or if he had a future at all. And so, he told his mother that he didn't think he was going to make it. He had serious reasons to believe that.

During his first hospitalization with pneumonia, doctors placed Weston in an isolation ward, which was a common procedure for dealing with AIDS patients, to prevent the disease from being spread, because at the time experts were not sure of all the ways it could be transmitted. When it came to HIV/AIDS, in order to follow hospital rules, both medical professionals and visitors had to go through two separate doors and a ventilation system to enter the patient's room.

Kurt Weston woke up hooked to tubes and machines, not sure what was happening to him. He opened his eyes only to realize that people wearing masks, gloves and suits were staring down at him.

During his hospitalization, doctors started him on intravenous Bactrim, a full-spectrum antibiotic used to treat PCP. The treatment started to work and a few days later Kurt began feeling better, well enough to sit in his bed with the IV medication dripping in his arm and watch the news on TV. That's how he learned that Queen's lead singer, Freddie Mercury, had just died of AIDS-related causes.

Unlike Mercury (who died of AIDS-related causes on November 24, 1991), Kurt Weston is still alive. The visual artist has survived his first bout of PCP and two others that followed. His doctor released Kurt two weeks later with a list of medications he needed to take as maintenance treatment and with a six-months-to-live prognosis.

Like Mercury, Kurt Weston was forced to keep his disease a secret, at the time. Kurt's physician advised him that the best thing for him to do was to continue taking his medication as prescribed and go back to work. He also advised Kurt not to mention to anybody at Pivot Point about his diagnosis, in order to avoid the stigma associated with the disease, because, the physician added, "people wouldn't understand [the AIDS situation]."

Once out of the hospital, Kurt followed the doctor's advice and took his medication—Bactrim tablets—to keep his pneumonia in check. He was also eager to resume whatever normality of life and career were possible. Yet, the process was a long and strenuous one, partly due to the virus ravaging his body and partly to the side effects to the very medication supposed to keep him alive.

In 1987 the FDA approved the first anti-HIV medication, azidothymidine [AZT], which had powerful negative side effects. While the drug was suppressing the replication of HIV, it was also causing bone marrow suppression that could lead to anemia, hair loss or a decrease in white blood cells. Other side effects included nausea, muscle weakness, and headaches. But AZT was the first AIDS medication to offer patients a sliver of hope for survival, no matter how slim that was. So Kurt had no choice but to take the drug if he wanted a chance to stay alive.

AZT made him extremely fatigued, to the point that Kurt started to find it more and more difficult to maintain the high energy level he needed to sustain at his job. As a fashion photographer he had to work with many people, from hair stylists and make-up artists to fashion designers, who were looking up to him to make decisions. It was his job to keep them motivated and enthusiastic in the studio, but in order to do that Kurt needed to be energetic and enthusiastic himself.

And all he wanted to do was crawl up in a corner, somewhere where everybody would just let him be with his fatigue, nausea, and sickness.

While that was impossible, the photographer had to gather all the energy he had left to keep up with the disease process, the medications and their side effects, and also to maintain an artificial version of what he was able to do and the perfection everyone expected of him. The entire process exasperated and exhausted him.

While Bactrim was an effective medication for keeping PCP in check, it wasn't unusual for patients to become allergic to it. When that happened, doctors tried to give patients other medications, but too often the results were not as effective.

Halfway into his treatment, Kurt experienced an allergic reaction manifested through rashes and fever. He became allergic to Bactrim and his doctor had no choice but to take him off the drug and switch him to something else. Kurt ended up trying several other medications, as the physician was trying to find one that would work at least as good as the Bactrim initially did.

One of the PCP prophylaxis treatments the doctor tried on Weston was pentamidine. The medication could be administered intravenously, intramuscularly (both used today to treat acute cases of PCP), or inhaled as an aerosol, which was later approved as PCP prophylaxis treatment.

While the intravenous pentamidine could cause severe pancreatitis, Kurt's doctor decided to start him on the aerosolized version and administer the medication as a fine mist the patient had to inhale. Kurt had to sit at a "machine" and breath in the mist containing the medications. He was doing this during his lunch breaks. But despite his doctor's high hopes, the treatment didn't work. The photographer ended up in the hospital, again, with a second bout of PCP.

By then, a new AIDS pneumonia drug, Mepron, was becoming available. Since 1991 Mepron has been approved for treatment of mild to moderate cases of PCP in patients who cannot tolerate standard treatments. Yet, when it became available, Mepron was only recommended for acute cases of PCP and doctors were not sure if it worked as prophylaxis. Besides, there were no instructions or guidelines regarding how to administer the drug; therefore doctors had no choice but to experiment with it and guess on the prophylaxis doses.

Kurt started to take a third of what was a regular dose of Mepron. Unfortunately it didn't work as expected and a couple of months later he ended up back in the hospital with yet another bout of pneumonia

Around that time, the photographer started putting his time and energy into reading as much as he possibly could about the disease, trying to find a way to survive it. That's how he came upon a San Francisco publication called BETA. The Bulletin Experimental Treatment for AIDS published an article that explained how patients could be desensitized, or adapted, back to Bactrim, while restarting them on the medication in small, pediatric doses. Excited about the new possibility, Kurt shared the news with his physician and begged him to try the procedure on him. But the HIV specialist thought the procedure was too risky.

In retrospect, the photographer believes today that any doctor would have reacted the same way because there was just not enough information about AIDS to allow these kinds of risky decisions from medical professionals. But that didn't mean that doctors gave up on their AIDS patients.

Several drug combinations later, Kurt's physician still couldn't find something that would work effectively on his patient. And it wasn't long until the doctor slowly started to run out of options when it came to finding new available medications that could keep his patient's AIDS pneumonia in check. He had one more choice left to help treat Kurt's PCP. That was intravenous pentamidine, a drug that could cause serious side effects and could increase the chances of developing pancreatitis. But the doctor tried it on Kurt and the treatment eventually worked and helped the photographer get over his third bout of PCP.

Out of the hospital for the third time, Kurt and his doctor had, again, to decide on a prophylaxis treatment. And again, Kurt pleaded with his doctor to desensitize him to Bactrim. This time the doctor agreed to it. The procedure worked and Kurt won another small, yet important battle with his AIDS.

By then, though, he had only three T cells left. Today, almost two decades into his living with AIDS, when talking to students about HIV/AIDS as a Positively Speaking volunteer, Kurt Weston calls his three T cells "the three Stooges: Moe, Curly, and Larry."

Yet, in the early nineties, Kurt's almost non-existent immune system was no laughing matter. His surviving was a paradox in itself, proving how strange AIDS could be and the various ways the disease evolved and manifested in different individuals.

When it first appeared in the U.S., AIDS seemed to have come out of nowhere—one day everybody was fine, and then, all of a sudden, people started getting sick, and dying, and disappearing. That's pretty much what was happening in Kurt Weston's life and in his friends' lives while he was attending school at Columbia College, pursuing his second Bachelor's degree, this time in photography. That made him a few years older than the rest of his classmates, and so it wasn't unusual for students to look up to him for advice.

One of these students looked up to Kurt for more reasons than just his seniority. Rudy was just realizing that he was gay, something Kurt had known of himself at an early age and never found it necessary to keep secret. Rudy was aware of that and looked up to Kurt to guide him through his coming out process. In time, the two became good buddies and started having lots of fun together. They remained friends even after their graduation from Columbia. But then things started to change.

Rudy, just out of the closet, immersed himself into the wild gay lifestyle of that time, trying to make up for lost time. He became solely interested in having fun, dancing and going club crazy. It didn't take him long to become a dancer at the Limelight.

The trendy nightclub is built within the shell of a stone, gothic style, old church building. The music is loud, the dance wild and people hot. But not everybody is allowed inside. Hired guards posted outside the nightclub get to pick and choose those who look hot enough to be allowed inside the club's sanctuary.

Limelight is an amazing place with a very long history, including parties, drugs, drinking and sometimes well-publicized scandals. A lot of the parties organized at these clubs went underground because the police were constantly watching.

Some people may find it strange about a church being a disco, especially those raised in a strict catholic tradition. Those who've worked at the club as club promoters or event organizers for years on say that surviving working at Limelight for three months is the equivalent of having a master's degree in club promoting, because working at Limelight is hard life and one had to be really dedicated and know exactly what one is doing.

Located in cities like Chicago and New York, Limelight is usually described as a place beyond one's imagination, where people come up with the wildest ideas, especially while on drugs. That's how they came up with the club dancers, or what they called "club kids," who were dressing up in outrageous and crazy costumes, and dancing in the club in suspended cages, or they were posing as live mannequins behind glass windows. "It was really weird, like a freak show," Kurt Weston recalls. "And Rudy became the ultra club kid who would dance inside a cage and everything."

In time, Rudy became quite a known person in the nightclub scene, but he continued to do it without Kurt, who lost interest in that kind of lifestyle. After a while, the two lost touch.

Kurt used to run into his friend every now and then. Later on he found out that Rudy was also slowing down and that he had a steady lover and settled down. And while Rudy's lover was pretty well off, the couple purchased a large industrial loft space, which Rudy eventually turned into his studio. And since his real name was Rudolpho, he called his studio Photography by Rudolpho. In a relatively short time, he started making a name for himself and doing financially well as a commercial photographer in Chicago.

While Rudy's photography business continued to soar, Kurt's workload at Pivot Point became overwhelming. He had asked Pivot Point to hire him an assistant. He even had someone in mind for the job—a young photographer, named David, with dreams of becoming an established photographer, and who was also very much aware that Kurt had specifically asked for him to be his assistant, thus offering him a first chance to jumpstart his photographic career.

Only two weeks after the young assistant came onboard, Kurt started getting very sick and ended up in the hospital for the third time that year with his third case of AIDS pneumonia. At the time, he was working on one of the Design Forum projects Pivot Point puts together each year.

With Kurt in the hospital and no other fashion photographer to take his place and finish the required photography, there was no imaginable way for Pivot Point to complete its trademark fashion book on time. So, Design Forum producers called Kurt in the hospital and asked him if he knew of any photographers who could just jump in and finish the project for them.

Kurt thought that Rudy could help, and so he called his friend and explained the Pivot Point situation. He told Rudy that he was very sick in the hospital, but said nothing about his AIDS.

Rudy accepted the challenge and went in and finished the job for Pivot Point before deadline. Design Forum producers were ecstatic about the results. They called Kurt to let him know about the wonderful job Rudy had done for them, how wonderful a photographer he was and how great it all worked out and that the book came out just perfect. And from his hospital bed, Kurt was happy for their success.

Right after his first hospitalization, the photographer had started visiting the local AIDS service organizations like Test Positive Aware, attending various meetings and workshops, and even seeking advice from TPA professionals, while still working full-time at Pivot Point. After Kurt's third bout of PCP, his case manager at TPA went against the doctor's opinion and told the photographer that it was time for him to leave his day job and apply for disability. "How are you gonna keep working, after three cases of pneumonia and only three T cells left?" the case manager asked Kurt.

But while the photographer realized that he couldn't continue working if he wanted to stay alive and a step ahead of his AIDS, he also didn't think he could leave work. The very idea of leaving the safety net of regular paychecks that assured him a comfortable existence was a scary thought. The very idea of his inability to continue doing his job was unimaginable to him. It meant that he was leaving his life up to hazard, especially at such a crucial time, when the disease was impairing his daily existence. How was he going to pay his loans, his bills? How was he going to pay for his treatments and medications? And what was going to happen with his health insurance he so desperately needed to stay alive?

Kurt had plenty of questions and no answers. Fortunately, his case manager started helping him understand what was going to happen to him while transitioning to disability and afterwards. The case manager explained that Kurt was going to have disability insurance and keep his benefits, and that he was able to survive even without a regular job. COBRA was to overlap the timeframe between his insurance with Pivot Point and Medicaid, but it could take up to eighteen months for the disability insurance to kick in.

Test Positive Aware helped Kurt with this transition. It also opened a door to Kurt's new community—the AIDS community.

Weston left work in 1993, finally realizing it was time for him to move on. And while starting his long and exhausting transition into living on disability, he secretly hoped that Pivot Point would hire Rudy to take his place.

During his third hospitalization and afterwards, when he was out on disability, Kurt continued to stay in touch with his young assistant. The photographer felt bad for leaving David to learn the job on his own and from Rudy through their work together on the Design Forum project for Pivot Point.

And also David stayed in touch with Kurt, calling him every once in a while to ask him questions regarding work or just to say hello and ask how he was doing. Therefore there was no surprise when, three or four months after he went out on disability, the photographer received a phone call from his former assistant.

"Have you heard about Rudy?" David asked.

Kurt, who was very sick at the time and pretty much confined to his bed, had no clue of what David was talking about.

"Rudy died," David continued. "He died of AIDS."

The news left Kurt speechless. He'd been hiding his own disease from Rudy and from everybody at Pivot Point for quite some time.

When he received David's phone call, Kurt was running fever constantly and battling cytomegalovirus [CMV] in his esophagus and eyes. Purple Kaposi's sarcoma [KS] lesions were starting to appear on his face and body. Rudy, on the other hand, had always looked great and never showed any signs of the disease noticeable on him. Yet, Kurt was still alive, while Rudy was not. That's what the photographer calls "strange" to this day.

Through the years, AIDS has remained a strange disease, touching people's lives in the strangest of ways. As an artist, Kurt Weston has used art as a means of expressing his own vision of the disease.

In that sense, Dark Angel may best capture Weston's first intimate experience with AIDS. The photograph is one of his first to be inspired by Angels in America, the play he went to see when it came to Chicago.

In Western monotheistic religions, angels are pictured as God's messengers, living among humans and in the transitional space between Heaven and Earth. They can be guardian angels helping humans throughout their physical life, or they can be angels of death, delivering the coming of Death. The concept of angels and the symbolism of funeral rituals concur in the artist's work, revisiting old concepts about life, death and the vast beyond that follows.

Kurt Weston's Dark Angel is an angel of Death. He is also an angel of AIDS, which, at the time, was a Death sentence. Weston's angel appears out of the shadows with his wings spread wide. The image shows actually an implied representation of the angel's wings, which are basically the shadows from where he's peering out.

Although the photograph is a mixture of poor light and shadows, the angel's face is clearly illuminated because, even if an AIDS prognosis meant a terrifying death, to the artist there's also something transformative about the disease. Throughout the years, AIDS has transformed many people's concepts about death and dying and about how people celebrate their lives and how they honor their dead. [Hence, the funeral scene in the 2003 movie, Angels in America.]

Before the arrival of the AIDS epidemic, many envisioned funerals as horrifying events where people would mourn and sob over an open casket. As the epidemic started to decimate the gay community and people started losing so many friends to the disease, funerals became more celebrations of life. And this transformation started to spread throughout the culture.

Weston's Dark Angel symbolizes an angelic figure composed of a play of the elements often used in the artist's work—darkness and light—to manifest the subtle interaction between what's real and what is not. This interaction further transposes between the dark angel and the white cat that doesn't seem afraid of the angel, but rather interested in his stake. The cat was actually "a happy mistake," the artist explains, talking about the technical part involved in creating the image.

The photographer used a view camera, which is a large camera that requires a piece of film, called sheet film, inserted in a film holder. He put this sheet film in the back of the camera and had the subject standing as he appears in the photograph, holding on to his stake.

The room was completely dark, as the artist started walking around the room with a handheld flash, popping the flash off in different angles to create different shadows as he walked around, thus creating the shadowy wings of the Dark Angel.

Unbeknownst to Weston, while he was moving around and working on his photograph, his cat, Che (from Che Guevara), walked inside the room and was accidentally illuminated when the flash came off. It wasn't until during the developing process that the photographer discovered the cat, which wasn't supposed to be in the picture, staring straight at the angel's stake.

Although Kurt Weston created Dark Angel in total darkness, he also interjected the only light into the image to illuminate the angel's face. The light is a symbol of hope and of life's triumph coming through the immense blackness of the (then) terrifying AIDS epidemic.

Balance

(For Kurt)

Angels and Demons,

Saints and Sinners,

Modern crucifixes,

Stigmatizing Life and what follows it,

Our Journey through Darkness and Light

And the shades of gray in between,

Matter and Antimatter

Make us whole and leave us empty

Creatures of a dual nature:

Surrenders and Survivors,

Warriors

Seeking a balance

In a world disturbed by shadows.

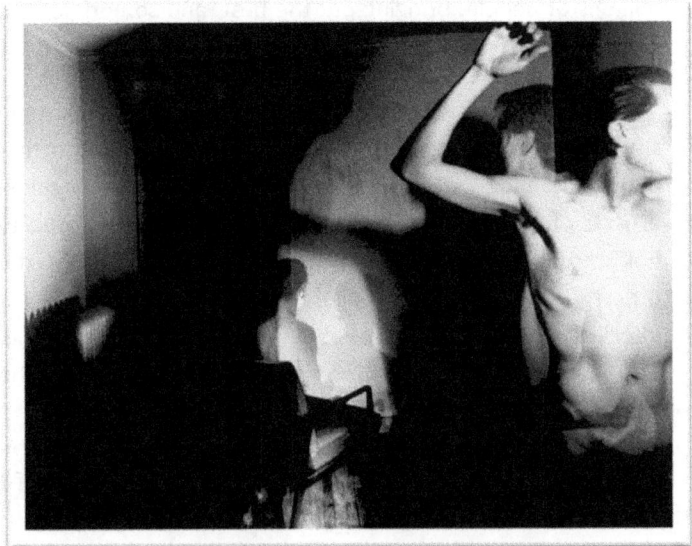

Chapter Four: Self-Reflections

Searching for Strength Within

AIDS is a puzzle of shadows, of darkness and light. It is hope in spite of suffering and forgiveness despite loss. AIDS is about duality—stigma and compassion, complacency and awareness. AIDS is about solving a multitude of issues, from medical and political to economical, social, and also human that have decimated communities and plagued countries and continents, leaving no oases.

AIDS has also changed people's attitudes toward life and death and the vast beyond that follows the physical dimension of human existence. The virus has touched tens of millions of people, bringing out the best, and sometimes the worst in its victims.

Kurt Weston believes that any kind of extreme situation, be that a disease, war or natural calamity that people are put in, can bring out the positive or negative aspects of their personalities. In the case of AIDS, this duality holds true for those living with the virus, and also for the others. There are times when some individuals who are not infected consider themselves above the virus and the disease. They see AIDS as a punishment sent by God to those who deserve nothing better.

The truth is that AIDS is a very human disease caused by a very human virus—the Human Immunodeficiency Virus. Since its worldwide outbreak in 1981, HIV has been perpetually mutating, transforming, hiding and disguising itself inside and on the bodies of those it has infected. Yet, the related stigma and prejudice, the isolation and fear always associated with the disease have stood the course of time. Something else that has been forever associated with this disease has been the mark (or stigma) it puts on its victims. This is only one aspect of what we've learnt to know as "the face of AIDS," and its persistent and perpetual transformation. One has to be a warrior to survive something of this magnitude.

In its early days, the psychological and physical burdens the epidemic brought to patients yielded to destructive, negative behaviors in some individuals. Faced with an imminent death sentence, some of those infected developed a "screw it all" attitude, and went on maxing out their credit cards and living totally irresponsible lives because they knew they were going to die soon anyway and didn't mind leaving somebody else to clean up their mess at the end.

Other AIDS patients did just the opposite. They became more responsible for their own lives and for the lives of those around them.

Kurt Weston met these kinds of people when he started attending AIDS-related workshops at some of Chicago's AIDS service organizations. Test Positive Aware was the first ASO he visited. TPA provided a helpful resource and a link to professionals who could help Kurt with his health insurance and medications, and also provide informative AIDS education. The organization also became a means of communication between the artist and others who were also infected.

At the time, the photographer was still recovering from his first bout of PCP and was very much aware that he should have been dead. And while he was still alive, he was uncertain as to how much longer he had to live... or how.

Being advised by his doctor to keep his disease a secret, there weren't many people he could talk to, openly, about his situation. But as he started frequenting, and later participating in TPA workshops and meetings, Kurt discovered that he was not alone. He discovered that other TPA members were going through situations similar to his, struggling to survive their opportunistic infections and fight their disease. They were HIV positive or had AIDS, in the early or advanced stages of the disease and, while around them, Kurt didn't have to hide his disease anymore. He also didn't have to explain how he had gotten infected, or why, or to come up with some excuse for his having AIDS.

While at Test Positive Aware, the photographer found one particular person went out of his way to try to comfort him for the simple reason that, at the time, this individual was himself going through the same process Kurt was, trying to recover from PCP, and, therefore, could truly understand what the photographer was going through. One year later this person became the executive director of Test Positive Aware. Within yet another year he died of cytomegalovirus, or CMV, in his gastrointestinal track.

It was also at the same AIDS organization that the photographer met other supportive people who had survived the tragedy of AIDS. They took the time to talk to him and to assure him that AIDS didn't have to be a death sentence but rather it could become a manageable disease. They were the AIDS survivors, living proof that what they were saying was the truth. And while he wasn't ready to give up on his life, Kurt became interested in finding out more about how these individuals could survive something as tragic and as deadly as AIDS. He became interested in discovering what kept them alive and what was the source of their hope, of the energy that was helping them maintain a positive perspective in life.

So, Kurt joined their group and listened to what they had to share. And their AIDS success stories touched his life in the most positive way, fueling his own desire to survive the disease. In time, the photographer got to know these early-AIDS survivors better and discovered that they were the ones willing to go the extra mile doing whatever it was necessary to fight the virus that was destroying them.

To this day, Kurt Weston considers these kindred souls his guardian angels, his first contact with the early AIDS warriors he later met in his life. They helped him take his first steps toward surviving the disease, while injecting in him a belief system that he, too, could turn his fate—his AIDS—around and transform it into something more manageable, into something that did not necessarily have to be a death sentence.

But learning how to stay alive required the photographer to take on some responsibilities of his own, including devotion and commitment to his life, and also a lot of time, money, and effort. These were the bases of living in a "surviving mode," which meant focusing solely on living one day at a time, while slowing down his life to bare necessities in order to stay alive.

A situation as extreme as a terminal illness forces individuals to stop and take time to relearn how to stay alive. Such an extreme situation starts by depleting individuals' existence one layer at a time until reducing their lives to basic surviving needs.

AIDS, for example, isolates and stigmatizes its victims, while taking away their social life, their connection with their families, friends, and peers. But it doesn't stop at that. AIDS continues by peeling off layer after layer of one's life, until there's nothing left. While the network of familiar faces (friends and family) may vanish first, the financial layer comes next. Patients are left jobless. With their bank accounts depleted, some are forced to live on disability. AIDS also attacks the most private layer of human existence, that related to the self-images individuals reflect on themselves and on others. The disease mutilates the physical appearance of its victims to such extent that it can permanently fracture this aspect of patients' lives. The intimate connections, the physical touches people need especially when during tough times, disappear shortly afterwards. And so do the personal and sexual lives of AIDS patients, because nobody desires them and nobody wants to be with someone whose body is deformed or who's sick and dying.

The actual physical death happens only after a slow and painful process during which patients are forced to experience the death of several dimensions of their existence. Those who manage to survive are sometimes left with virtually no means to do so; they are forced, therefore, to come up with their own ways of staying alive. Some do that by developing their own survival skills, like learning how to live in the moment or informing themselves about AIDS and researching various ways to stay alive even if only for a while longer. After all, they have nothing to lose.

Through it all, staying alive becomes an art in itself. Learning this complex process is not easy and not everyone has the kind of strength or inspiration required to attempt it.

More than fifteen years after his AIDS diagnosis, Kurt Weston considers himself lucky to have connected with people who could help him quickly learn how to fight the disease, and who gave him the hope and strength necessary to keep focused on his surviving. The photographer believes that being around survivors at that stage in his life and his AIDS was a vital part of his winning the battle with his disease.

While frequenting Test Positive Aware, Kurt was also completely taken by surprise to come face to face with people he'd known for a long time, in his pre-AIDS diagnosis existence. And he could read the same surprise in their eyes. And although it was obvious, everyone would inquire what the other was doing at TPA, yet no one was willing to say anything more or tell the true reason behind their presence inside an AIDS service organization building.

"Even in the gay community, if people knew you were infected, you were damaged goods," Weston explains. "[They] didn't want to have anything to do with you. It got so bad that friends I was going clubbing with, their first question was 'are you feeling ok?' or 'have you been feeling all right?'"

In general, people were attracted to the fun, the parties and the beautiful individuals attending these events. Nobody wanted to have to deal with other people's burdens, especially when associated with HIV and AIDS. So, Weston and others like him didn't really share their AIDS diagnoses with just anybody, but rather with only a few of the closest friends. It was a strange and at the same time sickening thing to do, but they had to constantly be aware of the aura of stigma and prejudice surrounding AIDS and those infected.

By the time he started frequenting Test Positive Aware, the virus was already starting to take a toll on Kurt, physically and also psychologically, depleting him of energy and vitality. Soon he became too sick to go out with friends and to handle the nightlife anymore, with its dancing, crowds and continuous partying. So, it wasn't long until he started losing contact with many of the people he used to know and go clubbing with.

In order to stay alive, Kurt started focusing his complete attention on getting over his opportunistic infections [OI], taking his medications, attending TPA support groups and listening to AIDS survival stories that were fueling him with the hope he needed to learn the survival skills, himself. At some point, when he eventually started feeling better and believing that he wasn't going to die the next day, Kurt realized that he needed to start putting his life back together, one layer at a time, until, hopefully, he could reach some sort of normality in his life or come as close to it as he could. And with each layer he was adding back to his existence, Kurt was getting better at surviving. In time, he began living again. He could then share his own AIDS survival stories with other members of his community and guide those who needed help.

Kurt also realized that he needed to add yet another layer to his life, one of physical intimacy. By that time his health recovered enough to allow the craving of some sort of physical contact and the company of another human being.

But dating, even within the AIDS community, was a challenge. There were disparities within the community between people living with HIV and those who had AIDS. Most of the time, members of one group didn't want to mingle, or have anything to do for that matter with members of the other group. An HIV positive person would not date or desire having any intimate connection with a person having AIDS. Even within the AIDS community, people wanted to know, firsthand, the stage of the disease of a potential date before actually making the effort to get to know that person better.

***

In 1993, after Kurt Weston went out on disability, a whole cascade of AIDS opportunistic infections started ravaging his body. His immune system became so deteriorated that purple blotches of KS lesions started to cover his face, body and his insides. At the same time, CMV continued to spread, attacking and scarring his retina and carving holes in his esophagus and creating enough damage for his doctor to wonder how Kurt was able to still be standing.

But he was still alive. If AIDS was to kill him soon, the photographer didn't want just to hang around waiting for death to come and take him. He was determined to fight until his last breath, so he started to search for new ways to stay alive.

That's how he found out about other AIDS organizations, like Northside HIV Treatment Center and AIDS Alternative Health Care Project. He started frequenting these ASOs too, and met people who were experimenting with alternative and Chinese ways of treating HIV. They were looking for unconventional ways to help them survive because too many of them had bad reactions to AZT.

Kurt also noticed that these individuals were not sharing their experiences with anybody. They would only whisper about their results with trying things like acupunctures, massage, yoga or the more drastic ozone treatments or drinking their own urine and other similarly bizarre therapies.

Their keeping secret this kind of information intrigued Kurt. He became interested in learning more about the various ways that could keep him—and others like him—alive. The photographer also realized that he needed to find a way to bring together those experimenting with alternative treatments to allow them to openly share their experiences with the others, so that everybody would become more aware of all possible ways to fight the virus.

So, in 1993, Kurt Weston founded SWAN. Surviving With AIDS Network was a grassroots group that met twice a week for one or two hours. Afterwards people could hang around to socialize and ask more questions. SWAN offered a safe place for people living with the virus to exchange their AIDS survival stories and experiences, no matter how extreme or bizarre they were.

For instance, because many AIDS patients experienced wasting syndrome and their bodies were losing muscle, becoming frail and with a skeleton appearance, Kurt invited nurse practitioners to his SWAN meetings to monitor the amount of muscle mass of the participants. It was a trade-off between patients and nurse—patients would go and help medical professionals in clinics and in return they would get a free BEI or Bio Electric Impedance test measuring their amount of muscle mass, thus monitoring the wasting process caused by AIDS.

Kurt also brought in medical doctors to talk about the latest medications coming up the pipeline. That's how SWAN participants found out about the life saving HAART (or Highly Active Anti-Retroviral Treatment) regimens, the protease and entry inhibitors that started to be FDA approved only years later in the mid-nineties. That's how SWAN members and participants learned about the upcoming drug called Fuzeon, which was FDA approved only in 2003. The entry inhibitor, supposed to keep HIV from entering (and then destroying) the T cell, took forever to hit the market because it was a complex drug that was extremely difficult to manufacture. Fuzeon is now available only as an injection. Twenty years and counting after being diagnosed with AIDS and over ten years from the founding of SWAN, Kurt Weston made Fuzeon part of his drug regimen.

One of the doctors who volunteered speaking at SWAN was an HIV specialist who was in particular dedicated to his work. Kurt noticed that the doctor was truly paying attention to his patients, treating not only the disease, but also the person it touched, and that he had an extensive knowledge of HIV/AIDS and was always on top of the latest, cutting edge treatments. The only way Kurt could explain the doctor's dedication, understanding and knowledge of the disease was to think that he was an HIV patient himself. In time, the physician became a regular at the SWAN meetings.

Kurt was so impressed with the doctor's willingness to try treating AIDS with some of the most aggressive treatments available at the time that he decided to become his patient. After his third bout of pneumonia, the photographer saw for himself just how open his new physician was to experimental treatments—his new doctor was the one who agreed to desensitize Kurt back to Bactrim. A couple years later, in 1995, when Kurt left Chicago and moved to California, he left his physician to take over the SWAN meetings.

Before the advent of HAART regimens, a lot of the disease progression depended on the patient's immune system. For example, the kind of opportunistic infections, how long these O.I.s would last, how well the medications could keep the infections in check or how fast KS lesions (that appear in the advanced stages of AIDS) would appear or disappear.

"The first time I noticed a [Kaposi's sarcoma lesion] on my body, it was kinda on my wrist," Kurt recalls. "All of a sudden I saw this purple blotch on my wrist." He looked at it and wondered if he bruised himself somehow. But when he went to the doctor, he found out it was Kaposi's sarcoma.

Then, all of a sudden, KS lesions started coming out all over his body. Kurt had the cancerous purple blotches on his face, nose, legs, down his throat, on his chest and his back, on the roof of his mouth and also in his esophagus.

Looking back, the photographer finds it now odd that long before he even knew he had AIDS, every time he was going to his dentist for regular cleaning and check-ups, the dentist kept mentioning that there was something strange growing in Kurt's mouth, something that shouldn't have been there. At the time, the photographer had no idea what the dentist was talking about. He had no idea that his mouth was full of thrush, which, in those circumstances, was a sign of AIDS. But the dentist should have known, especially when his office was located in a part of Chicago with a predominant gay population and especially considering that he had a lot of gay patients. Yet, the dentist only told Kurt that he had some kind of fungus in his mouth, not calling it thrush, not really calling it anything and not giving his patient any advice.

While at Test Positive Aware and while holding his SWAN meetings, Kurt seemed to be in the advanced stages of AIDS, battling KS and other opportunistic infections. Sometimes patients needed chemotherapy or radiation to get rid of their KS. Kurt's doctor decided against chemotherapy for his patient because the treatment was extremely immune suppressive and Kurt's immune system was already extremely weak. The physician opted for radiation to treat the lesions only on Kurt's face because an individual could cover everything else but his face. And in case Kurt wanted to wear shorts during the summer, his doctor also agreed to radiation of the lesions on his patient's legs.

Kurt was to see a radiologist whose office was located in the same hospital his doctor was practicing. The radiologist checked out the lesions and agreed that radiation could help get rid of them. The only side effect was that the areas on the face treated by radiation would become very dry, years later. "But you see these symptoms happening to people twenty years down the line," Kurt remembers the radiologist saying, "and you're never gonna live that long to see [this happening]." To this day, the photographer still recalls the blunt words, said in a matter-of-fact voice.

Obviously, almost twenty years later, Kurt Weston continues proving him wrong. But at the time, the grim future the radiologist sketched out for him shocked the photographer, and the physician's comment and attitude freaked him out.

Yet, he ended up going through several radiation sessions. During one of the sessions, the doctor radiated his left eye. At the time Kurt also had molluscum contagiosum warts on his left eyelid, which the doctor thought it was a KS lesion and that radiation might help.

***

Molluscum contagiosum is a skin disease caused by molluscum contagiosum virus, or MCV, which can be transmitted from person to person. MCV is also autoinoculable, meaning that the infected individual can transmit (or spread) it to himself. The MCV infection is generally characterized by small bumps that appear on the face, upper body, or extremities. MCV infects mostly children and adults with impaired immune systems, the latter experiencing the viral infection manifested as tiny, pearl-like papules on their face. When the T cell count falls below two hundred, as it happens in AIDS patients, the lesions start to spread.

Kurt Weston experienced MCV and the KS lesions at the same time on his face. Molluscum contagiosum virus felt like pebbles stuck under his skin that he spread on himself every day, when shaving. So his entire face became covered with warts. He had them around his eyes, on his nose, his cheeks and down his neck. And it looked unimaginably horrible. "I would walk out and people would look at me like 'oh my God, what's wrong with this man?'" the photographer recalls. "It was horrifying. I looked like a circus freak and it was very devastating to me."

Kurt's doctor sent him to a dermatologist who was nice, but who mostly treated teenagers with pimples on their faces. The specialist had never before treated the kind of disease Kurt had, but he did his best.

He explained to his patient that there were two ways to treat the warts. One involved freezing the warts with liquid nitrogen and the other, dabbing them with a blistering solution. The dermatologist was skeptical using liquid nitrogen on his patient's face because it could cause scarring and discoloration, so he advised to go with the blistering agent.

The substance used in the procedure was extracted from a blister beetle carrying the chemical in its body. The dermatologist was to dab Kurt's warts with the solution, which, in turn, would cause the warts to pop. Then the blister would heal and the warts would go away. Kurt thought about it and decided to go with the blistering agent.

The dermatologist then told his patient that he was going to cover only twenty warts at a time because the procedure was going to be "really hard" on Kurt. So the doctor took what looked like a long toothpick, dipped it into the blistering solution and started dabbing some of the warts on his patient's face, and then let him go home.

Once out of the doctor's office, Kurt met one of his friends and together they went shopping. While in the store, he started feeling something really itchy on his face and while he couldn't see his own face, his friend could. "Oh my God, Kurt," the friend said, "your face is turning into a huge blister!"

The two of them ran out of the store as fast as they could and headed to Kurt's place. Once inside, the photographer rushed to the bathroom and stared at his reflection in the mirror. His face looked like one of a burn victim. Blisters had filled up over the warts and literally popped with fluid, and there was also a bit of blood gushing out of them and of his face. It also hurt like hell... so bad that at night he couldn't turn his face on the pillow.

Kurt had to go through several of these sessions for almost one year. During this time, KS lesions and MCV warts covered his face. While Kurt didn't want to leave his home looking like that, he had no other choice, because there was nobody else there to do the shopping and run the errands for him. The sad part was that the warts went away right after the treatment but once the skin healed, new warts grew right back. They seemed to never go away entirely and it took an endless battle to get rid of them. It was debilitating for Kurt and, sometime in 1994, he decided he couldn't continue the treatment any longer.

***

While under radiation therapy, the specialist who was treating the KS on Kurt's face thought that the wart on his eye, large and reddish as it looked, was also a lesion and that radiation would help. But while the specialist couldn't just radiate the patient's eye, he covered it with a lead plate, which looked like a very thick cup with a handle sticking out of its center, so that the doctor could stick it on the eyeball and then pull it off. It sat on Kurt's eyeball like a suction cup to prevent it from being radiated.

The doctor radiated Kurt's eyelid several times and actually got rid of the MCV wart that way. But the procedure also damaged the photographer's eyelid so that it could no longer produce tears for the eye to stay hydrated. [Lachrymal glands are located above each eyeball and produce tears, which are then spread over the eyeball by blinking.]

Kurt's left eye, with a damaged lid, started getting dry and scratchy. Its lashes fell out and when they started growing back, they grew back all crooked, like whiskers, scratching his cornea every time he blinked.

They felt like sand in his eye and he had to go to the doctor every two weeks to have his eyelashes plucked. Each visit lasted three hours or so, because he had to spend a lot of time in the waiting room. That was until Kurt had enough and asked his doctor to find another solution to his eyelid.

So the physician came up with the idea to make a cut into Kurt's eyelid and stitch the eyelid up, so that the lashes would grow up and wouldn't scratch his eye anymore. And Kurt thought it was a good idea, so he allowed the doctor to go through with the procedure. But as it turned out, the surgery shortened Kurt's eyelid so that it couldn't close fully anymore, thus not allowing his left eye to stay hydrated.

Years later, after CMV retinitis left him totally blind in his left eye, Kurt decided to use an eye patch, which also keeps enough moisture in the eye. Ever since then, even after he couldn't use his left eye anymore, Kurt has continued to care for it daily, applying lubricating gel to keep the dryness out and wearing the eye patch twenty-four hours a day.

***

The appearance of KS lesions on Kurt's body was a sign of the advanced stage of his disease. Yet, Kurt was lucky. His lesions didn't hurt. They were discolored and very unattractive, but because they were dry, doctors could treat them with radiation.

Other patients were not that lucky. Their lesions were fluid-y inside and would burst out and hurt. For these patients, therapies like chemotherapy or radiation were not always possible and they had to walk around and go out in public wearing their lesions on their faces and their bodies, carrying with them the grim—purple, in the case of KS—flag of AIDS, exposing themselves to being pointed at and even further stigmatized and discriminated against. Therefore, many people with KS lesions refused to go out anymore and became prisoners in their own homes with their disease.

In 1993, when Kurt and other people attending SWAN meetings were battling KS on and inside their bodies, Philadelphia had just been released and become quite a hit. So those who'd gone to see the movie thought they learned a lot about the differences between a birthmark and a Kaposi's sarcoma lesion. To this day, the photographer cannot watch the movie past one of its early scenes, when AIDS-stricken Andrew Beckett (played by Tom Hanks) covers his KS lesion on his forehead when his boss asks him if that was a birthmark... So, especially after the release of Philadelphia, people with KS lesions on their faces could not show themselves in public without being identified as having AIDS.

Weston was one of these people that the epidemic was threatening to confine to their homes and isolate from the rest of the society. And Weston would not accept that. There had to be a solution to this situation and the photographer felt compelled to do something about it, to regain his—and others'—freedom to go out and about their businesses and be able to show their faces in public without fear of stigma or judgment.

While at Pivot Point, Weston had worked with many make-up artists, so he called up some of them and asked them if they could help. They showed up at his SWAN workshops and offered make-up sessions, showing participants what kind of make-up to use that worked best with their faces, how to use the make-up to look most natural and how to best cover their KS lesions.

Soon, the word went out and traveled across Test Positive Aware and other similar local organizations, and more people started to show up at Kurt's workshops. So many of them, in fact, that they needed to bring chairs from all over the building to accommodate everybody. After a while, Kurt even had to ask for a larger room that would fill, each session, with seventy or eighty individuals.

During 1993 and 1994, while Kurt continued to monitor his SWAN workshops in Chicago, people would attend for a while, and then some of them would just quit coming. They were either too sick to leave their homes or already dead. It was typical for those attending AIDS support groups to see individuals participating and talking to others during the meetings and then disappearing, like they've never existed. And it was very frightening for the rest of those attending and trying to survive the disease... Years later, this real-life aspect of AIDS support groups was forever immortalized in the Broadway musical—and later on movie—RENT.

While the conventional medicine didn't have much to offer at the time and the only treatment available was making them extremely sick and weak, people living with the virus were desperate to try pretty much anything that could remotely improve their quality of life, and they would listen to anybody who could possibly offer them a chance to survive. AZT was a first positive step toward finding an AIDS treatment, but not all patients could manage staying on the drug.

A lot of them felt so sick while taking the medication that they quit caring about living. If the drug, which was supposed to keep them alive, made them feel so awful, what was the point of being alive in the first place. Some would rather be dead and end the suffering altogether.

Other patients believed in a conspiracy theory, that the Big Pharma (the large network of drug companies) was trying to make money off AIDS patients and that the chemicals in the AIDS drugs were poisonous and doing them more harm than good. So a lot of infected people refused to take the AZT or go through chemotherapies. They attempted a more natural approach to fighting their AIDS.

A lot of those attending SWAN workshops also became extremely interested in alternative treatments. Therefore, a lot of alternative medical practitioners showed up at SWAN meetings to inform the patients of other ways they could fight the virus.

"There's a lot of fakery in the world of alternative treatments," Weston explains. "And some practitioners were preying on people with life threatening, terminal illnesses. [But] if some [medical] doctor came to you and said that you were gonna die because you had this [disease] and there was nothing available to help you, and then somebody else came and said 'I know something that they don't know. I've got this thing that could help you.' Wouldn't you be tempted to try it?"

During the SWAN meetings alternative medical practitioners showed patients how to keep themselves healthy using therapeutic nutrients, Chinese herbs, and acupuncture. They also discussed very extreme therapies like Ozone therapy, auto-urine therapy or the benefits of various plant extracts and enzymes. That way, patients could get a better understanding of the various possibilities available— other than just chemicals—to treat their HIV. That way, AIDS patients could become more proactive fighting their disease.

Alternative treatments were very expensive and patients who wanted to try them couldn't afford to try every one of these treatments. Most of the patients were on disability and didn't have much money to spend on experimentations, even on those who could potentially extend their lives. In addition, it would have been very time-consuming, plainly not smart and simply not possible for each individual in the SWAN group to experiment with every one of the available alternative treatments.

So, SWAN participants decided to take turns, and then get together and share what worked and what didn't work. If it worked, than it was worth the money. If not, then the others didn't have to give it another thought.

Each member of the SWAN group volunteered to try various things. For example, one person would take herbs, another would attend an acupuncture session or try urine therapy, while yet another individual would go through a session of Ozone therapy or take yoga classes or massage therapy sessions. And regardless of their experiences, either if they found them helpful, successful or just plain gross, participants would come back to the following SWAN meeting to discuss and share their trials and thoughts with the rest of the group.

Weston himself has tried some of the most extreme treatments. "I did try drinking urine," the photographer confesses. "Because one of the Chinese medical practitioners said that some people got very good results from drinking their own urine... so I did that. And I don't believe that it really did work, but I was willing to try anything."

***

Drinking one's own urine is also known as auto-urine therapy, uropathy, or amaroli. Before being used as a treatment, amaroli began as a spiritual practice used by yogis of old times to purify their bodies in order to allow the consciousness to expand to its original, cosmic state. In present society, amaroli has re-emerged as an effective alternative therapy used worldwide.

For internal use, individuals can drink from one to three glasses of their urine per day. Conditions and optimal use may vary if drinking the urine is done while fasting. Midstream urine should be sipped like tea. For external use, individuals can rub their urine on cuts and bruises.

***

In the case of AIDS, the theory behind this "treatment" was that the urine contained dead viral fragments that, if re-ingested, could help the immune system, just like taking an attenuated virus and emulating one's immune system to attack the virus.

The whole concept made Kurt vomit. He describes the experience as "horrifying." But on the other hand, the urine was free and he had nothing to lose.

Another alternative treatment SWAN members tried involved a substance called Carnivore, extracted from the Venus Fly Trap, or VFT, the only carnivore plant in the world.

Like humans, the many varieties of VFT plants are genetically different from each other. VFT has very thick, fleshy leaves, or petals, with traps (or "teeth") at their end. The plant can create a red pigment in its tissue, which is supposed to attract the insects (some experts believe that it is also used to protect the plant from sunburn). When a fly lands on it, the petal closes and kills the fly with its "teeth," and then digests the fly with the help of an enzyme within the VFT plant.

The theory was that this particular enzyme, the juice within the plant, could help treat HIV. The enzyme would digest (or disintegrate) the protein in the HIV, and therefore destroy the virus. Patients could buy it from a company in Germany and they could give themselves Carnivore shots intramuscular or intravenous... so Kurt did both.

Another treatment he also tried required injecting himself with a substance called Iscador. Ten injections cost eighty dollars. Iscador was a therapeutic homeopathic preparation created from mistletoe, a very poisonous plant, which is fatal if ingested.

But the mistletoe story doesn't start with AIDS or with Christmas. In ancient times, pagans in Northern Europe held orgies before mistletoe altars. This reverence translated into the Christian ritual of hanging mistletoe over doorways at Christmas time. The pagan orgies became, through the years, the custom of kissing under the mistletoe.

Mistletoe is a parasitic plant that grows in the bark of trees and does not obey many of the laws of the plant kingdom—it stores up chlorophyll and stays green throughout the year, indifferent to light. The name "mistletoe" comes from a Celtic word meaning "all-heal," thus its historical use as remedy for pretty much everything from nervous complaints to bleeding wounds and tumors. Many years later, traditional Chinese and Korean medicine discovered a variety of uses for mistletoe.

In the early twentieth century, Rudolf Steiner, the creator of anthroposophy (a human oriented spiritual philosophy) introduced the plant to modern medicine. He used medical mistletoe, called Iscador, as a potential cancer treatment and mistletoe extract injections as immune system stimulants.

***

While at SWAN, Weston hasn't tried only the extreme treatments, the Iscador and Carnivore, but also therapies like acupuncture, yoga, meditation and massage, which enhanced his inner strength and gave him new hope that he would survive the disease. Through this kind of gentle treatments, the photographer met wonderful people who offered him the spiritual support he needed to get through that stage in his life. They stood by his side when the PCP, KS and CMV were ravaging his body and they helped him come through.

These alternative therapy practitioners did not dress like regular doctors. The photographer remembers his Chinese acupuncturist looking like a witch doctor, a Bohemian, wearing wild clothes and carrying with him various herbal preparations. He used to put needles in different parts of Kurt's body… like the voodoo with his voodoo dolls.

During his first visit, the acupuncturist did an analysis on Kurt, placing three fingers on his wrist to take his pulse—that was the photographer's energy pulse or "chi"—which measured the essence of life flowing through his body. The acupuncturist then told Kurt that his chi was really strong, thus making Kurt feel that he had enough life force to survive the disease.

Most of the volunteers donating their time and kindness to organizations like Test Positive Aware were not infected, yet they were not afraid to work with infected people, to talk to them and comfort them, to touch and hug them, give them massages and embrace them with their bodies and their spirits. To this day Weston thinks of these volunteers as being "the best of humanity."

One particular lesbian woman, called Hannah, was what Weston considers his first "warrior." She took her philosophy from the Native American culture. She was teaching tai chi and yoga classes at TPA because she believed in the power and benefits of moving energy. Hannah believed that one's physical body can be controlled by one's mental attitude, and that by combining the power of one's mind with the power of one's will, a patient could affect the outcome of the disease process.

Hannah would end her yoga class by doing a relaxation exercise where she would team up students and have them massage each other so that they could be relaxed and meditative. One time she teamed up with a man whose face and body were covered in very severe KS lesions. Anybody else would have used rubber gloves before touching the poor guy, but not Hannah. She did not hesitate massaging and relaxing him, and was not afraid to touch his lesions. She was completely fearless, inspirational, and motivational.

And for Kurt she was a tremendous inspiration in strengthening his survival instinct. It was through Hannah that the photographer realized that there were people who could create an inspirational energy in others, and who could give others hope.

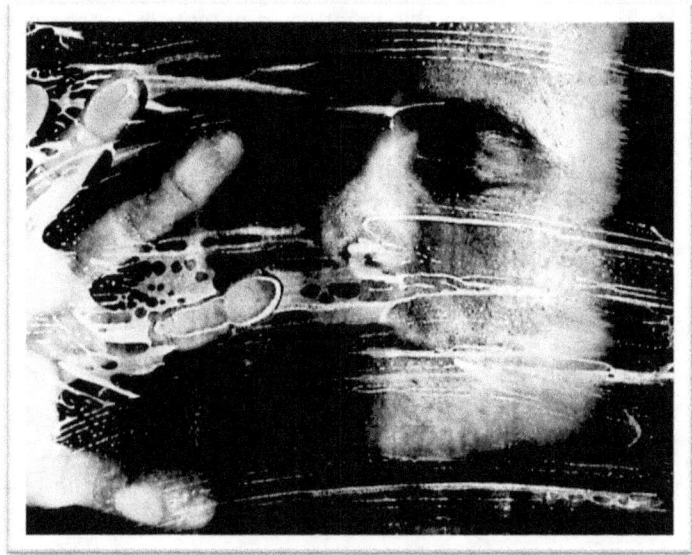

Chapter Five: Losing the Light

"Cotton in My Eyes": CMV Retinitis

By the beginning of 1994, when snow was still covering the ground, purple KS lesions were covering Kurt Weston's face and body. They were definite signs of the deteriorated state of his immune system. He had spent months going through several radiation treatments for the lesions on his face and legs, but the Kaposi's sarcoma kept coming back and his AIDS kept progressing.

With no cure in sight and no life-extending medications available at the time, the photographer and many others living with AIDS became increasingly desperate to try just about anything that could potentially extend and improve their lives. While conventional medicine offered only a mono-therapy their bodies could barely manage, many AIDS patients turned to unconventional ways to care for their disease. Some have even experimented with a few of the most extreme alternative treatments like ozone therapy, which the photographer, himself, decided to try.

**

Ozone is a gas discovered in 1839 by a German scientist named Christian Friedrich Schonbein. The name "ozone" comes from the Greek "ozein," which means "(to) smell." Its molecule is relatively unstable and of a pale-blue color (which gives the color of our sky). Ozone is formed when ultraviolet light or an electrical discharge splits an oxygen molecule into two highly active oxygen atoms. The recombination of atomic oxygen with the oxygen molecule that follows forms the tri-molecular oxygen, called ozone. The gas has a bleach-y like smell that is sometimes felt in the air after an electrical storm or in the vicinity of electrical equipment.

A gas like ozone, with such a simple molecule, turns out to have quite some dramatic effects on life on Earth. In the higher layers of Earth's atmosphere there is what scientists call "good ozone" because it protects life on Earth from outside ultraviolet radiations, and also people from getting skin cancers, cataracts or impaired immune systems. Closer to the Earth's surface, where the gas comes directly in contact with human life, there is what experts call "bad ozone," a harmful pollutant that can damage the lung tissue. This "bad ozone" is also a major constituent of smog.

Ozone can also be used in oxygenation (or oxygen) therapies—a type of alternative therapies said to cure cancer or impaired immune system related diseases. The seeds of the oxygenation therapy concepts are found in the works of William F. Koch (1885-1962), a Detroit physician, and Otto Warburg (1883-1970), a researcher and double Nobel Prize winner—once in 1931, for discovering the oxygen-transferring enzymes in cellular respiration and again in 1944, for identifying the enzymes that transfer hydrogen in metabolism.

Oxygenation therapy has many pros and cons and the definite disapproval of the conventional medicine experts. Oxygenation therapy proponents explain it as being based on the presumption that a deficit of oxygen in the tissue (also known as hypoxia) can cause human disease and, therefore, lead to immune system's failure to kill invading bacteria and viruses. An infusion of pure oxygen (like ozone) can restore this function of the immune system.

There are two substances usually recommended in oxygenation therapy—hydrogen peroxide and ozone. Their names determine the type of oxygenation therapy.

Originally discovered in 1818, hydrogen peroxide is a substance present in nature in trace amounts. It decomposes violently when it comes in direct contact with organic matter. Light, chemicals like carbonates, proteins or chlorides are only a few factors that can accelerate the decomposition of hydrogen peroxide. Therapy using a "food grade" (thirty-five percent) hydrogen peroxide solution suggests that patients should drink the substance, use it for brushing their teeth, for soaking in a bath with it or massaging it into their skin. Patients can also use it as douches, colonic irrigations or intravenous infusions.

Ozone can also be used in oxygenation therapies intravenously, intramuscularly or as colonic irrigation. During the early nineties, some of its proponents advertised that ozone therapy could cure AIDS by inactivating extra-cellular HIV. And either they believed that or not, AIDS patients were willing to give it a try.

**

To receive the treatment, Kurt Weston had to travel to a small town outside Reno, Nevada. His father ended up going with him because patients were advised to have someone by their side, while taking the ozone.

The therapy lasted ten days and cost fifteen hundred dollars. While patients kept pouring into the clinic, seeking hope and survival, doctors practicing conventional medicine were advising against such treatment, warning individuals that they could die of aneurism. But as far as Weston knew, nobody died of aneurism while or after going through ozone therapy.

Ozone therapy isn't, by any means, a cure for AIDS but, as the theory goes, it has the potential to improve a patient's immune system. The gas is administered using an ozone generator. It has a pungent odor that can affect the sinuses and can produce choking if inhaled. Weston remembers instances when patients at the Nevada clinic were playing, blowing ozone on latex gloves and then watching how the gas literally shredded the glove into pieces.

On Kurt's first day at the clinic, a medical doctor inserted a PICC line into his vein, at the bend of his arm, through which to administer the required daily dozes of ozone. It took the doctor three minutes to insert Kurt's first ever PICC line. The procedure was painless and the photographer didn't even have time to realize what was happening to him.

*****

A PICC line, or Peripherally Inserted Central Catheter line, is a thin flexible silicone tube that medical professionals insert into patient's vein and through which they administer intravenous medications, transfusions or chemotherapy for long periods of time. This way, the patient doesn't have to make frequent hospital visits to receive necessary treatment or to be given multiple injections. For optimal results, the PICC line has to reach the large veins in the patient's chest. This allows medical professionals to administer large amounts of medication directly into the bloodstream. Therefore, the medications can work fast and most efficiently.

Nurses are usually the ones to start the PICC line. They can insert the tubing straight in the patient's chest using general or local anesthetic. In this case they call the line a central line. Nurses can also insert the tubing in the patient's arm, usually near the bend of the elbow, and in this case the line is called a peripheral inserted central catheter line, or PICC line. After starting the PICC line, nurses then use an x-ray machine to help them guide the tubing all the way up into the patient's large veins in order to make sure it is in the right position (close to the heart). Only then can they begin administering the medication through the PICC line. The entire procedure requires only local anesthesia of the skin where the line is inserted and it generally takes about thirty to forty minutes.

***

The medical personnel at the Nevada clinic used the PICC line to administer the ozone. What followed was a hellish ten-day therapy that Kurt was determined to survive. "You get high fevers and your teeth are clutching," the photographer recalls. "You start shaking [until you] feel like every muscle in your body starts knotting up, like getting into convulsions."

Those who worked at the clinic prepared heated blankets to wrap around the patients to keep them from shaking. After completing the daily ozone sessions at the clinic, patients were taking ozone containers with them to the hotel where they were staying during the ten-day treatment. While in the hotel room, they had to pump the gas into their rectums.

During therapy, Kurt got hallucinating fevers of a hundred and four degrees. He became sick, enough to worry his father, who tried to convince him to stop the treatment altogether and go back home to Chicago. But Kurt refused to give up and insisted on finishing his therapy. And when he did, he saw his T cell counts soaring.

This gave the photographer some hope. He even came up with the idea of purchasing a small ozone generator and continuing his treatment at home. The only problem was that he didn't have a PICC line in his arm anymore. The doctor at the Nevada clinic had taken out the tubing from his arm once he was done with his ozone therapy. The only other way he could self-administer ozone was to self-inject with the gas… but that was something he did not believe he was able to do.

Yet, the ozone home therapy opportunity was far from vanished. During the following years, between 1994 and 1996, the photographer was to go through some twenty-five PICC lines that medical professionals had to insert in and take out of his arms to administer intravenous ganciclovir medication for his CMV retinitis. Later on, he used those PICC lines to self-administer his ozone, using a home ozone generator that he ended up purchasing after all.

***

Cytomegalovirus, or CMV for short, is a herpes kind of virus that infects most adults, especially after a certain age, and is transmitted in many ways, including eye contact with unclean hands. Once the virus enters the person's body, it stays there for the rest of that person's life and most of the time it doesn't cause any damage. People in normal health are usually unaware of having it.

When the immune system starts deteriorating below a certain level (T cell count becomes lower than fifty, measured per unit of blood), CMV becomes active and can attack various organs, like the lungs, esophagus or the eyes. When the virus infects the lungs, it causes CMV pneumonia. In the eye, the virus attacks the retina causing CMV retinitis, which, if left untreated, can lead to partial or total vision loss. CMV retinitis is the most common cause of blindness in people living with AIDS.

With the advent of HAART regimens in the mid-nineties, the number of cases of CMV retinitis in people with AIDS has decreased by ninety percent because the new medications keep patients' immune systems strong enough, with T cell counts way above the fifty count limit, thus not allowing favorable grounds for CMV activation. [Appendix B: CMV at a Glance deals with CMV retinitis in more details.]

***

Kurt Weston's vision loss didn't happen overnight. The photographer experienced the first symptoms of CMV retinitis in 1993, while he was still working at Pivot Point. When preparing the room for a photo shoot, he would notice flashing spots on his backdrops or he would see shreds of cotton and start blinking, trying unsuccessfully to get rid of them. Only later he realized that those shreds of cotton floating in his view were floaters and one of the first signs of cytomegalovirus attacking his eyes.

Although Kurt always kept his doctor's appointments and went for his regular checkups, his eye specialist kept misdiagnosing him. A few years later, in California, his new doctor determined that the virus had been doing extensive damage to his patient's eyes. Parts of Kurt's retina had been infected and then healed, while other scars on his retina were more recent, together causing permanent damage to his sight.

The virus also spread to Kurt's esophagus. He started experiencing severe heartburn, so he went to see his doctor. An endoscopy showed that CMV had been making a huge hole in Kurt's esophagus, causing serious damage... enough to make the doctor wonder how his patient could still manage to walk around.

Kurt's first treatment for CMV retinitis involved a medication called ganciclovir. Twice a day, every day, a pump the size of a small tape recorder would administer the necessary dose of intravenous ganciclovir through a PICC line directly into Kurt's vein.

The actual process of inserting the line in Kurt's arm was extremely difficult and painful using a large needle that Kurt didn't think would fit into his vein. A nurse had to insert a yard worth of intravenous tubing in his arm, and then to guide it up his vein, all the way near his heart. An x-ray machine helped her monitor the entire process and the location of the intravenous tubing so that she could make sure that the line reached the large vein, where it needed to be for maximum infusion of the medication.

It so happened that Kurt's nurse was new at running PICC lines up patients' arms. The procedure didn't work as planned and so she had to try it several times. She failed each time. When she finally succeeded inserting the needle into Kurt's vein and started guiding the tube inside, the tip of the needle would hit the inside walls of the vein, causing him even more discomfort.

As the nurse was guiding the tubing, it eventually got stuck halfway up Kurt's arm. She tried to continue the procedure, but no matter what or how hard she tried, the tubing seemed to move no farther. Several failed attempts later Kurt started already to be in pain. He also became more and more exasperated with the entire procedure and the nurse's lack of experience. But the more exasperated he became, the less options she had to finish inserting the PICC line in his arm. So, she thought that it was best just to give up for the day. She rolled the remaining tubing under his arm and decided to administer the medication anyway. Then she left, telling Kurt that she was going to be back the following day to take the PICC line out and reinsert it in his other arm. And so she did, and the second time around she succeeded without any problems... and also without using any anesthetic.

Sometimes, while inserting a PICC line, the tip of the needle could "burst" the patient's veins. Some patients on intravenous medications experienced these "bursts." Their PICC lines cracked and scratched their veins, leaving bluish spots on their arms.

For the next couple of years, Kurt Weston has continued going about his daily routine, while having the tubing into his vein and the medicine pumping in his bloodstream to keep the CMV from further damaging his eyes. He has continued running his SWAN meetings, keeping up with his doctor's appointments and his medications.

He managed to stay alive. Yet, the PICC line interfered with every aspect of his life. Moving his arm up and down and back and forth caused Kurt's tubing to move and start coming out of his vein, a little with each move. Every time he had to take a shower, he first had to wrap a plastic bag around the external part of his PICC line and then secure it in place with an elastic band, to make sure it was safely covered so that it would not get wet.

Every so often, the nurse stopped by Kurt's home to change his tubing and flush the line through with sterile saline solution, but the photographer was the one who had to care for his PICC line around the clock. Therefore, he had to learn how to change his dressing, start the IV medication and do daily maintenance of his PICC line. The entire process was complicated and emotionally devastating for the photographer:

First, he had to make sure the boxes of PICC line kits were shipped to him on time, so that he would not run out of medication. Each of the kits contained everything necessary for him to start his intravenous medication—the hypoallergenic tape, the Betadine swab, the alcohol, bandage, cotton swabs and the boxes of syringes.

In order to start the IV, Kurt also needed the actual bags of fluid that came at a "mind-boggling" price. These bags of fluid needed refrigeration, especially during the summer, when temperatures soared over one hundred degrees. Therefore, during all the years of intravenous therapies, Kurt's refrigerator was constantly half-full with bags containing intravenous fluid, which, eventually, had to be injected in his body.

Once the yard-long tubing was in his arm and the IV running, Kurt had to keep his PICC line clean to reduce the risk of infection. Maintaining the PICC line required knowledge, patience, guts and daily attention. Yet, it could not guarantee to keep the potential infections at bay.

The whole maintenance process required tedious work and became an intrinsic part of Kurt's daily existence. Every day he had to clean the external part of the line to keep the tubing from getting stuck or infected. Every day he had to peel off his dressing, clean the skin around the PICC line with alcohol, put the Betadine bandage and then replace the dressing with a new one. And each time he peeled off the dressing, he'd have no choice but also pull a bit of the tubing out of his arm. After a while, the PICC line slowly started to migrate out of his vein, until it was out so much that it needed to be replaced. That's when the nurse had to come in to replace the tubing.

Kurt Weston has lived with PICC lines in his body and with bags of intravenous medication in his fridge for a couple of long years. During this time, nurses had to insert into and take out of his veins some twenty-five PICC lines, enough to make his arms look like those of a heroine addict.

One summer, when the photographer was really sick while living with PICC lines in his arms, a friend from San Francisco decided to fly in and visit. The photographer remembers him as a very self-absorbed man who was also living with the virus. He wanted to see how Kurt was doing, and also to visit Chicago and have some fun while in the city. Around the same time, another friend happened to be in town to visit Kurt. And so the three of them decided to go to Grant Park to a Bastille Day (July 14th) concert. But before they could leave, they had to wait for the nurse to stop by and replace Kurt's PICC line.

The day was humid and torrid, with temperatures soaring way above one hundred degrees. When the nurse finally showed up, she was already covered in sweat, which was rolling down her cheeks, neck and arms, sticking to her fingertips. She followed Kurt to his bedroom and got to work. As she kept trying and failing to insert the new PICC line into Kurt's vein, the friend who also happened to be in town stood by the photographer's side and held his hand. He could not ease Kurt's pain, but he could at least try to keep him calm and comfortable as much as it was humanly possible.

Meanwhile, on the other side of the bedroom door, the friend from San Francisco started getting increasingly impatient with having to wait on Kurt and his PICC line. The entire procedure was taking way too long and he was concerned he wasn't going to make it to the concert on time. So he started pacing the apartment, yelling through the closed door, demanding to know what they were doing inside and what was taking them so long. Yet, he never offered to help or to go inside and see with his own eyes what was going on.

By then the nurse was doing her best trying to stay calm and "cool" and to ignore the heat coming from outside and the angry voice outside the bedroom door. Unfortunately it wasn't helping her much. The harder she worked, the more she started to doubt her ability to get her job done. She began apologizing to Kurt, and it was Kurt who ended up comforting her, telling her that it wasn't her fault and encouraged her to give it one more try.

Throughout the entire ordeal, the friend by Kurt's side left the room only once, when he had enough of the whining coming from outside the door. He went to tell the other guy to leave and go to his concert, and that he and Kurt would catch up with him when they were ready. Then he resumed his seat by Kurt's bedside, as the other guy stormed out of the apartment.

It took the nurse three tries to get the PICC line in Kurt's arm. Afterwards he could again self-administer his medication and not worry about it for a while longer.

Living with the PICC line in his body was not easy. Kurt had to deal with the side effects to the medication and keep up with cleaning and maintaining the line. He also had to keep his PICC line from being noticed whenever he went out. He had to hide all the tubing sticking out of his vein for multiple reasons—to protect his PICC line from getting damaged, to protect himself from being stigmatized and judged, and also to prevent people from freaking out when staring at his arm.

Over time, Weston came up with various ways of camouflaging his PICC line. He would cut out the top of a gym sock and use it to cover up his arm, or he would buy one of the supports, the elbow braces, from a sporting goods store. Using the brace looked more natural, as if he'd had a sports injury.

Years later, when he moved to Orange County and was asked to speak to students about HIV/AIDS as part of Positively Speaking program, Weston would appear at the workshops wearing that sock to cover his vein. And while talking with the students about HIV, he'd pull the sock down and show his young audience his PICC line and explain how the medication was administered through that tubing in order to keep him from going totally blind. And while doing so, he'd notice some girls in the classroom turning ghostly white, although none of them really fainted.

Kurt did use his PICC line beyond administering conventional medication. Because his T cell count went up during his ozone therapy and as he now had the necessary means to self-administer the ozone, the photographer bought himself a home ozone generator and resumed his therapy. For one year or so, Kurt and one of his friends injected themselves with ozone. They used small doses in order to minimize the side effects as much as possible—that meant only ten cubic centimeter (cc) shots of ozone, six times a day, every day.

While Kurt's friend didn't have a PICC line, he begged and pleaded with Kurt to inject him with the gas and he didn't stop until, after much hesitation, Kurt finally agreed. The photographer continued using his PICC line until right after he moved to California, when his new doctors there took it out and talked him into trying other ways to administer his HIV medication.

***

In April of 1995 Kurt Weston received a phone call from his younger brother. The call was not a surprise, but the reason for the call was. His brother, who was living in Orange County, invited Kurt to move in with him. He knew how much Kurt loved the West Coast because the photographer visited as often as he could. So, his brother hoped that Kurt would give it some serious thought and accept the invitation.

Weston did just that and considered it an opportunity to start fresh. And so he began planning his move right away. He intended to have everything packed and the flight ticket in his pocket by the end of August. That way he had a full summer ahead of him to get ready for the West Coast.

Meanwhile, the ganciclovir medication administered through his PICC line and supposed to treat the CMV in his eyes has stopped working. As it happens with viruses (CMV and HIV included), they mutate a lot and become resistant to medication, thus forcing doctors to switch their patients to new drugs in order to keep the infections in check.

Kurt's doctor decided to put his patient on a new medication, called foscarnet. The problem was that foscarnet had several serious side effects, one being severe kidney damage. Therefore, before even being able to start the treatment, Kurt had first to receive infusions of pure saline solution to hydrate the kidneys and minimize the side effects to the medication. Several months later, the foscarnet treatment started to fail and CMV resumed attacking even more of Kurt's eyes.

This treatment wasn't the last of its kind that Kurt had to go through. The infusions required Kurt to stay hooked to an IV pole twelve hours a day. And while he could not do that, medical professionals administered the medication using a backpack and a small CADD pump—an electronic pump the size of a small walk-man.

During this kind of treatment, Kurt had to carry gallons of fluid medication in his backpack, hook his IV tubing into the pump and then turn it on. That way, while the device was pumping the medications hour after hour into his veins, Kurt could walk around, run his errands and his SWAN workshops, and keep up with his doctor's appointments and TPA meetings.

It was during one if these treatments that Kurt's PICC line got infected. It caused fever and fatigue, and it required antibiotics. If not caught in time, the infection could spread throughout the body, causing serious sickness and even death.

Meanwhile, the heat and the sweat of that summer did not help the infection to go away fast enough, yet Kurt managed, somehow, to get over it. Through it all, he continued sorting through his things, deciding what to pack and what to leave behind, getting ready for the West Coast. And while doing that, he also turned into a not-for-profit organization, putting together fundraising events to raise some money for his trip and for other post-Chicago expenses

While preparing for the move, Kurt sold or got rid of what he didn't need or what he couldn't take with him. He always had to think three times before deciding what to do with his things and what to take with him that could fit in the room his brother had offered him. And it was terribly hard for the photographer to decide because he didn't know how much longer he had left to live. Because he had no way of knowing if he was moving to California to start fresh or to die. "It's very hard when you're moving and dying," he explains. "And you get rid of things that are really meaningful to you, [of] part of your life."

That particular year Chicago went through a torrid summer. The heat wave claimed hundreds of lives and overwhelmed health officials. Morgues were overloaded and unable to accommodate the corpses that kept arriving at their doors. So, city officials were forced to put in place refrigerator trucks to store the bodies until the morgues could get them.

Kurt had a third—and top—level apartment and the temperature inside stayed steady at one hundred degrees despite the three air conditioning units and several fans that were constantly running. Stretched down on the floor, carrying his medication in his backpack, Kurt was trying to get everything ready for his move across the country. There were times when he thought he was going to pass out, when his heart started racing until it was almost impossible for him to breathe. There were times when he thought he was going to die of heat exhaustion.

But he survived and finished packing. And on September 4th, 1995, he got on the plane to California. It was Labor Day weekend.

The entire moving process had been intense, but Weston never regretted it because by the mid-nineties, he had no more close friends left in Chicago. They all had died of AIDS. He wasn't really leaving anything or anybody behind. Besides, despite the fact that he loved running SWAN, he was also aware that his health and his life at the time were not the best. He thought that, somehow, California would help. To this day, Weston believes that had he not moved from Chicago, his health and the overall quality of his life would have been much worse.

But the move to California was bittersweet. Three weeks after his arrival, Weston started to attend the local AIDS organizations in Orange County where he met new people and made new friends. Also, during his first months in California, the photographer became legally blind because of the experimental treatments his new doctors tried on him.

While in Chicago, he'd had to go through the daily hustle of maintaining the tubes sticking out of his veins and his arms, but in time Kurt started getting quite good at managing and caring for his PICC lines. Meanwhile, new treatments and new medications became available, and Kurt's new doctors in Orange County wanted him off the PICC lines. So, they persuaded him to try the new and improved ways of administering intravenous medications.

One procedure required doctors to surgically insert silicone gel implants in Kurt's body. The implants were called PassPort and were otherwise known as "implantable venous access ports." These new kinds of catheters were working pretty much like the PICC lines, only that the catheter was not visible outside the body, but it extended from the port to the large or central veins in the body. The silicon port could be accessed through a needle, and thus the medication could be administered through the needle into the port and farther on through the tubing and into the bloodstream.

The ports Kurt's doctors wanted to use on their patient were made out of metallic plates on top of which was a silicone gel hump (or septum). These ports were to be surgically implanted under the skin, in the muscle of the chest or arm.

The procedure sounded pretty straightforward to Kurt. In addition, using the new implants he wouldn't have anything dangling out of his skin anymore. So he agreed to have the small surgery done and opted to have the silicone gel ports put in his arm, because he didn't want anything implanted in his chest.

The procedure was done in October 1995, and right from the beginning the port became infected. Doctors put Kurt on antibiotics to subside the infection, but the treatment didn't work.

A month later Kurt was running a fever over one hundred degrees. He went back to the hospital where doctors found out that the infection was coming from a nasty bacteria stuck in the tube of the device underneath Kurt's skin. But while insisting that he needed to have the port in his arm, they did not remove it. Instead, they gave him a massive amount of antibiotics.

For the following three months, Kurt kept having very high fevers despite the oral and intravenous antibiotics he was on. He ended up being hooked to an IV pole all day long, with two daily infusions of antibiotics and two daily infusions of ganciclovir for the CMV in his eyes, pumping through his veins.

Yet, the antibiotics did not get rid of his infection. In addition, his T cell count dipped to almost null. With his immune system virtually non-existent, the ganciclovir also quit working, because the medication needed some immune system to act on. Therefore, Kurt's CMV retinitis started running out of control.

At this point, Kurt didn't care if he was to live or die. He didn't care if he was going to upset his doctors. He just wanted the device out from under his skin. The doctors finally decided to take it out. For that, he had to go through yet another surgery. The following day all Kurt's infections started to go away. But by then the CMV had already destroyed more of his retina.

By January 1996 the photographer started to realize that he was already legally blind, but when he shared his concerns with his doctor, the HIV specialist remained sure he could save Kurt's vision. The available solution was to try two new, experimental medications to treat the CMV.

About the same time a new life-saving medication was coming on the market. It was one of the first protease inhibitors (or P.I.s) medications called Crixivan, and it was part of a new treatment called HAART (pronounced like "heart") regimen, otherwise known as "the cocktail," which was going to radically change patients' lives, turning AIDS from a definite death sentence into the manageable disease that AIDS is today.

The Highly Active Anti-Retroviral Treatment was (and continues to be) a revolutionary triple-drug therapy made possible by Doctor Ho of the Aaron Diamond AIDS Research Center in New York City. HAART put Doctor Ho on the cover of Time magazine and made him Man of the Year in 1996.

These new kinds of medications first started coming out in December 1995, so during the previous months, drugs like Crixivan were still under last, or phase three, of testing and on the verge of getting FDA approved. Because there were not enough medications for everybody needing them, some drug companies offered to give them to patients on a compassionate use basis only, otherwise known as expanded access programs.

EAP was (still is) a program through which pharmaceutical companies distributed upcoming medications that were already in the pipeline but yet to be FDA approved to people who needed them most. This process had been very rare and extremely difficult before the AIDS years. Usually, a doctor had to call the manufacturer and then the FDA, fill out hours-worth of paperwork and wait for months to get a drug sample, enough only for one patient. And then start all over again, for the next patient. And so on.

Fortunately AIDS has changed all that. The epidemic has forced people living with the disease and AIDS organizations to learn fast the drug industry regulations, to meet with people from the industry and with government officials and to draw proposals. But nothing really happened until people living with AIDS went out in the streets and demonstrated, literally, for their lives. A familiar example is the 1988 ACT-UP demonstration on Wall Street, New York City. [ACT-UP, or AIDS Coalition to Unleash Power was founded in 1987 (www.actupny.org).]

Only then, the FDA started allowing drug companies to open trial programs as soon as they had available at least some safety information on the drug. That's how the "drug lotteries" started in 1989. There were several such lotteries and participants had to meet several criteria.

For example, in 1995 Glaxo provided a (then) upcoming medication called 3TC to over thirty-two thousand people in the United States. It was the largest expanded access program ever.

Merck announced its Crixivan lottery in July 1995. The company was giving away drugs to eleven hundred people in the U.S. and an additional seven hundred fifty patients from twenty-nine countries in Europe, South America, Canada, and Australia. Merck was to pay for the drug, including shipping, and also for post-selection central laboratory tests and the urine pregnancy tests when and if needed. To be able to participate in Merck-organized P.I. lottery, AIDS patients had to meet several criteria, including to be clinically stable, to be able to follow directions and have certain T cell counts and viral loads. [Glossary to this book provides more detailed information regarding definition of terms like T cell count and viral load.]

The lottery took place in August 1995. In Chicago, Kurt's doctor put his patient's name in the program. By December, Kurt's new doctors in California received a phone call from his former physician: Kurt had won the lottery. He was one of the eleven hundred AIDS patients approved to receive the new drug. Winning the drug lottery literally saved his life. To this day, the photographer seriously doubts his ability to stay alive if it wasn't for the new medication.

He started treatment in January, right before he got his doctors to take out the silicone gel inserts from his arm. At the time, there was no way for Kurt, or his doctors for that matter, to imagine the powers of the new HAART regimens, to think that in just a matter of months they would be able to bring his immune system back on track and far from the dangerous zone of CMV activation. All Kurt's physicians knew for sure was that if their patient didn't receive the two experimental treatments fast enough, he would lose his vision for good.

But Kurt knew that his vision was already gone. It took him several months to get his doctor to accept the truth. It wasn't until May of 1996 that the physician finally agreed to give Kurt a certificate stating that the photographer was legally blind. He needed it to register to the Braille Institute where he could learn how to survive in his new world of new insecurities, and darkness.

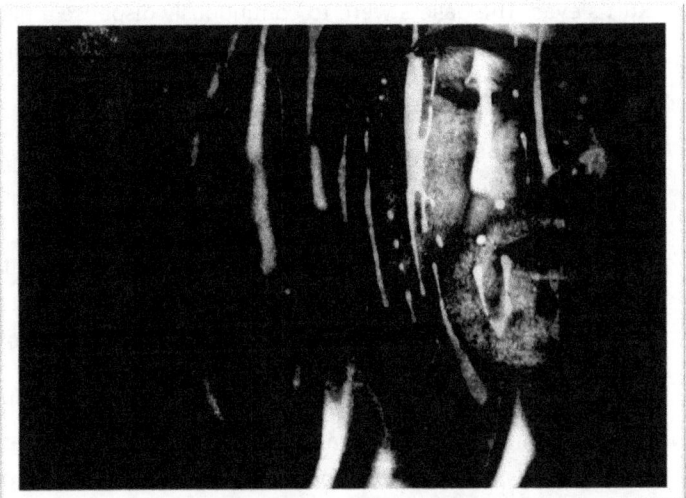

Chapter Six: Journey Through Darkness

Blind Vision

To this day, Kurt Weston still believes that had the doctors used only one of the two experimental medications, he would still be sighted. But, while his doctors, the HIV specialist and the eye specialist, could not decide which one was most critical to treat—the CMV in the photographer's esophagus or the CMV in his eyes—they tried to treat both infections simultaneously, using two powerful medications. And that turned out to be too much for their patient.

The first experimental treatment involved a surgery through which the eye doctor implanted ganciclovir pallets in

Kurt's eyes. The pallets were to continuously dispense a high amount of medication directly into his retinas, thus treating the infection in the fastest and most efficient way.

The second experimental treatment involved a medication called cidofovir. Administered every two weeks as intravenous infusions, it was supposed to treat the CMV in Kurt's esophagus and to prevent the virus from spreading to other organs. One year into the treatment, though, doctors started realizing that the medication was harming Kurt's eyes.

Being simultaneously administered directly into the bloodstream, the two medications completely overwhelmed Kurt's retinas, causing a complete annihilation of his central vision in his right eye—he couldn't focus anymore—and complete blindness in his left eye. As a result, the photographer became legally blind.

To this day, Kurt Weston continues to suffer from the outcome of the side effects to the two medications. Because of the new HAART regimens he's been on, CMV is not active in his body anymore, yet the virus has left permanent scars on the photographer's retinas. Therefore, his eyes need constant care in order for him to maintain whatever vision he has left. He has to use daily prednisone eye-drops (an anti-inflammatory steroid) that burn his eyes but also prevent further retina inflammation.

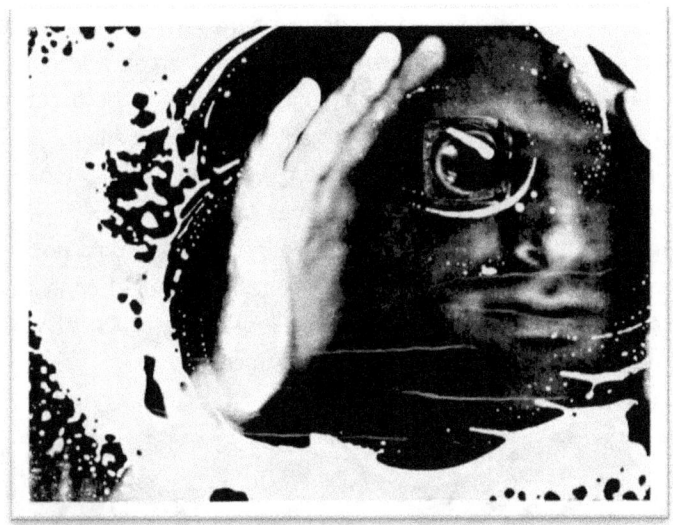

Peering Through the Darkness

Realizing the damage the experimental medications had done, Kurt's doctors apologized to their patient and had no choice but to admit their failure of saving his sight. Encouraging promises of earlier months turned into hopeless messages. Kurt was going to be legally blind for the rest of his life and there was nothing anybody could do for him anymore. Doctors could not give him his sight back and medications couldn't stop or reverse the infection progressing in his eyes. Life as Kurt knew it dispersed instantly giving room to a confusing and terrifying uncertainty. The photographer found himself isolated yet again, the way he'd felt when first diagnosed with AIDS, surrounded only by a hopeless and endless blackness.

"I was devastated because here I had spent my life working as a photographer and as a visual artist, and now I was no longer capable of doing this... or so I thought, because I couldn't see anything in focus," Kurt Weston explains. "For instance, if I were to be in a room with you, I would look at you and would not see your eyes, or your nose, or your mouth. I would see the tone of your skin, but would not be able to see you smiling, or frowning, or winking. I don't see anybody's face. I see... like if you look at the palm of your hand. That's what I see of a person's face."

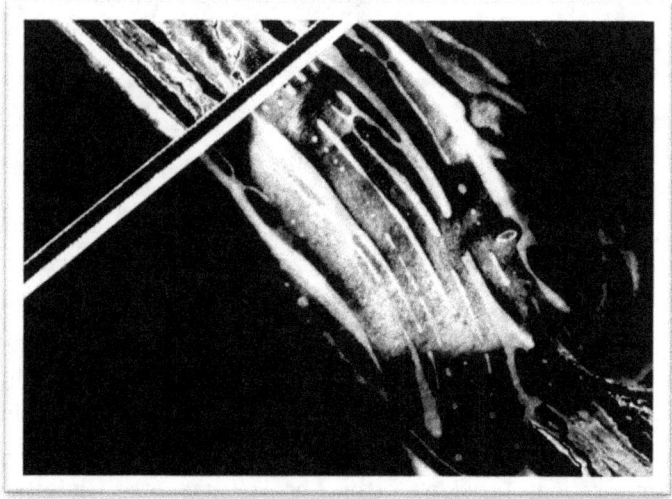

Blind Hell

Not long after his official diagnosis, Kurt talked to a friend and told him about his becoming legally blind. It so happened that the friend knew somebody who was working for amfAR in New York City, and so he offered to help Kurt.

He told the photographer that amfAR would be interested to hear his story and encouraged Kurt to call the AIDS agency.

Founded by Dame Elizabeth Taylor in 1985, the American Foundation for AIDS Research (amfAR) is one of the first of its kind. To this day, the agency continues to provide services and to advocate for people with HIV/AIDS.

Kurt took his friend's advice to heart and called amfAR and, indeed, those he talked to were really disturbed and upset hearing his story. But when they took action and called Kurt's doctors, both physicians had already changed their stories and blamed their patient's legal blindness on Crixivan, the newly FDA approved protease inhibitor medication that Kurt had just started taking only a month before deciding to proceed with the two experimental treatments. It wasn't until much later, when the possibility of a lawsuit was at safe distance once again, that the two doctors went back to their original opinion regarding the cause of Kurt's vision loss.

Confusion comes easy. So does self-destruction and self-doubt, especially in a situation like Kurt's was. It is often easy to get entangled in the debilitating game of questioning oneself and of judging one's actions. It is often difficult to stay clear of the multitude of "what ifs," "only ifs" and second-guesses threatening to redefine one's past. There were times when Kurt's own AIDS, and later on his vision loss, had threatened to push him further into this labyrinth of confusion, at times almost to a point of no return. Therefore, his secret for surviving had always been to never allow failures from the past to govern his life, to alter his future and keep him from making the best of his situation. He wasn't going to change that kind of guidance even in the face of his permanent vision loss. Therefore, the photographer pleaded with his doctors until he got the necessary paperwork to enroll in classes offered by the Lower Vision Department at the Braille Institute.

It was vital for him to start learning how to survive and how to "see" again in his new world, in order to move forward with his life and his dreams. Kurt had to start by learning how to use a cane, work with adaptive technology and read Braille. And he didn't have to do it all alone, because he had the support of his new partner.

Kurt had met Va Hong after moving to Orange County, while attending a Positive Friends meeting at one of the local AIDS support organizations. Va was a "wonderful Vietnamese man" whom Kurt found "very cute." The two started talking and found out they had quite a few common interests. It didn't take them long to start dating and afterwards to begin a serious relationship.

In time, as Kurt started losing his sight, Va became not only his partner but also his guide. Va ended up taking Kurt to his doctor's appointments, which were spread all over the city, and everywhere else the photographer needed to go. Va also introduced Kurt to the Asian Pacific Crossroads group, a local organization serving Asian Americans living with HIV/AIDS. There, Kurt got to meet many people who knew Va and form meaningful relationships. Va was the one to tell Kurt about the Braille Institute and encourage him to attend classes.

While the Braille Institute was providing useful information through hands on activities and courses, it also required students to live on the campus. And while Kurt didn't mind doing that, he really didn't enjoy his staying there either. To him, the Braille Institute looked more like a senior center. Most of the patients were in their seventies and eighties and most of them had lost their sight to age, to macular degeneration. To Kurt it seemed that they were only there to kill time, while he needed a fast and immediate immersion in studies that would allow him to continue his life despite his visual disability.

Besides, Kurt had different kinds of problems. He was the only one to have lost his sight to CMV. He was the only one who had AIDS. Yet, upon his acceptance, the Braille Institute officials instructed him not to mention his disease or the real cause of his blindness to anybody. "We just think it would be better if you don't tell anybody about your situation, because, you know, people don't understand," they told him.

The advice reminded him of his doctor's words years earlier, in Chicago, when he was working for Pivot Point and was recently diagnosed with AIDS. The officials at the Braille Institute listed Kurt's reason for being there as cystoid macular edema, which is a swelling of the macula, and which Kurt had as a result of the side effects to his medication that had damaged his macula, thus his ability to see things in focus with his right eye.

During his short stay at the Braille Institute, Kurt couldn't really connect to anybody or make any friends, so he tried to stay focused on his studies and relearn, as fast as he could, how to get around in his new world. He attended all the classes that were required of him, studied hard and learned quickly.

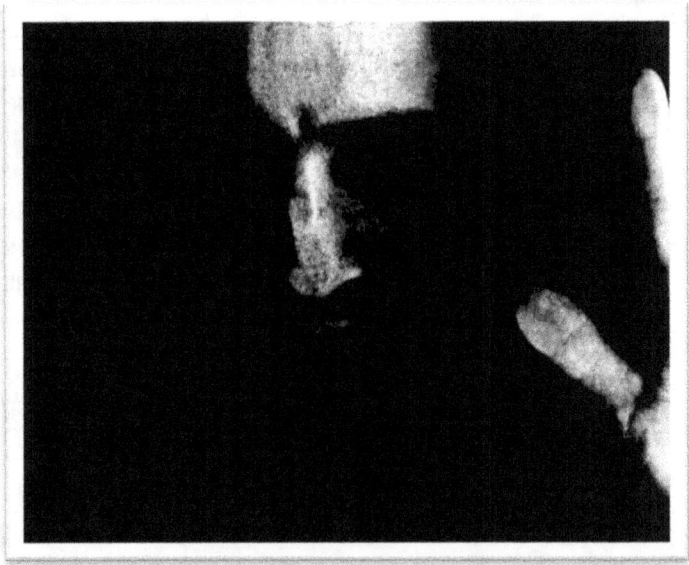

Requiem

One of these classes was a beginners typing course. The instructor suggested that it would be a good course for Kurt who, at the time, was not computer savvy. So the instructor set Kurt at the keyboard and started him on his typing. Moments later, the photographer found himself struggling to stay focused on what he needed to do. He tried his best to go through the course smoothly, but found it terribly boring. Yet, he kept typing the same letter over and over again before moving to the next letter and repeating the process. No matter how much he would try, Kurt was slowly getting bored out of his mind. So he started eavesdropping on conversations going on around him, which seemed to be much more interesting than typing letters ad nauseam.

That's how he decided that one particular conversation was, indeed, worth his undivided attention. Kurt overheard one of the seniors in the class talking to the instructor about his Department of Rehabilitation counselor, how wonderful she was and what wonderful things he had learnt there. From what he heard, Kurt realized that what the rehab program had to offer was just the perfect kind of low vision classes he needed, and he memorized the counselor's name and phone number, and made a quick mental note to contact her as soon as he could.

Later that day, right after he was done with his classes, Kurt made an appointment with the counselor. Not long afterwards she stopped by his place and explained everything to him about the program and all the benefits it had to offer. She also told Kurt about the Foundation for Junior Blind, describing it as offering similar courses as the Braille Institute, but at a more intensive pace.

To attend courses at the Foundation for Junior Blind, Kurt would also have to live on campus, in Los Angeles, during the week and then return home to Orange County for the weekend. And knowing that he eventually had to learn how to negotiate and live his life as a visually impaired person, Kurt accepted the challenge and started the long application process and the endless waiting period for an opening.

During the few months Kurt had to wait to actually start his studies at the Foundation for Junior Blind, his partner, Va, started to get really sick. Va was hospitalized with AIDS-related lymphoma and, because the pain was becoming more than he could possibly handle, doctors had to put him on morphine. It took Va a couple of weeks to die. He passed away on January 8th, 1998. And throughout the entire ordeal, Kurt has remained by his bedside.

Literally two days after Va's death, the photographer received a phone call from the Department of Rehabilitation. They had good news. There was indeed an opening available at the Institute for Junior Blind and they were waiting for him in Los Angeles to start his courses immediately.

But no matter how promising the opportunity, at the time Kurt found it impossible to make himself attend school. He wasn't ready just yet, not while he was still mourning the loss of his partner. Va's death had been slow and horrible, and Kurt had had to witness his lover's suffering and to live through all the pain and loss that came with Va's passing. The experience had left Kurt numb and overwhelmed by a sorrow he didn't know how to escape. So, while risking what could have very possibly been his only chance to relearn how to "see" again and get acquainted in his new world, Kurt politely declined the offer and was ready to give up his slot.

Fortunately, the Institute for Junior Blind rep on the phone with Kurt wasn't as eager to let him give up. While there was no telling when the next opening was available, she recognized that Kurt's situation was indeed special and offered to hold the slot for him for another two weeks, while making him promise he would think about it and call her back.

Reserving the spot was a difficult task in itself, especially when so many people were waiting in line to enroll in the classes and Kurt was very much aware of the favor she was doing him. So he did think about the journeys to come in his life. He wouldn't have been able to learn about the Institute for Junior Blind if he hadn't gone to the Braille Institute in the first place. And he had been able to do that because of Va's encouraging him to move on with his life. So, two weeks later, Kurt called back the institute in Los Angeles and told them he was ready to start his studies.

The photographer also realized that he needed to get away in order to break away from the memory of Va's death. He needed to go to Los Angeles and learn to negotiate his life again, to find his way around and to function in his new and still unfamiliar world.

Because Va was not there anymore, Kurt had to learn how to get around on his own. While there was no way he could get around the town on foot, he had to renegotiate his transportation and he had to do it fast, because he couldn't afford to miss his doctor's appointments if he wanted to continue living and staying ahead of his disease.

The photographer found out about a local transportation company called ACCESS, which was serving disabled people. The price was reasonable and the service reliable. So Kurt arranged for ACCESS buses to pick him up from his home, drop him where he needed to go, and then take him back home. He also ended up using ACCESS to commute between home in Orange County and school in Los Angeles.

Despite the hard work and difficult schedule, Kurt enjoyed his studies. He had great instructors and learned how to work with adaptive technology in order to make use of computers. He also learned various other helpful things that could help him get started in his new life. Learning to read Braille was one of these helpful things, but nowadays Kurt is the first to confess that he's never been good at it because he's never been able to really feel the Braille dots due to the AIDS-related neuropathy (numbness) in his fingertips.

While at school in L.A., Kurt also learned how to use specialized programs that allowed him to magnify the letters and words on the computer screen as much as necessary for him to read his emails and documents. Zoomtext is such a software program that has a "Document Reader" function that reads the text back to Kurt in a woman's (or male's) voice, depending which one he chooses.

The photographer impressed all his instructors by excelling in all his courses and graduating from Institute for Junior Blind in only half of the time usually required to complete the course. Only three months after his enrollment, Kurt Weston received the certification to prove that he was ready for the road ahead.

While still in L.A. and halfway through his studies, Weston had the chance to reconnect with the Asian Pacific group and its members he'd met through Va. The experience turned out to fulfill one other legacy Va had left him.

One Valentine's Day weekend in 1998, Kurt had just gotten back home from school and was looking forward to some much needed rest, when a few members of the Asian Pacific Crossroads group called him to invite him to a party. At first, Kurt declined the invitation. He was too exhausted and had a full week worth of studies in Los Angeles ahead of him. But the Asian Pacific members refused to take no for an answer, and even offered to pick him up from his place and take him to the party. So Kurt accepted to go with them in the end.

It was at this party that the group organizers decided they wanted to raise money for the organization through a fundraising project—a calendar featuring some of the Asian men who were members of the organization.

"All we need is a photographer," they said.

"Well... Kurt is a photographer," the ones who knew Kurt pitched in.

"Yeah, but I'm legally blind now," the photographer said.

They were somehow disappointed and asked him if he'd ever tried to photograph after losing most of his sight. He still had his equipment, but couldn't see anything clearly, so he wasn't sure he could even focus the camera anymore. They interpreted his insecurity as hope and decided to give him two models to practice with for the calendar pictures and see what he could do.

So, he ended up using his special equipment, the handheld telescope and special magnification finger-thick glasses he'd purchased with the help of the Department of Rehabilitation. Kurt worked with the two models for a full afternoon, using different lighting for different pictures. The process was much slower than when he used to work as a fashion photographer.

At the end of the photo shoot, Kurt presented Asian Pacific Crossroads with a few sample photos of his models and waited for their reaction. And they took a look at his work and were amazed by its quality. They named him their photographer and decided to let him shoot the entire calendar.

Kurt Weston started to work on his project in May of 1998, and while doing so he began to learn—and then to master—the use of his special equipment. The learning process didn't happen overnight. It took time and patience. The photographer had to work much slower and make sure that everything was in focus, although sometimes he couldn't be certain. It took him months to finish the 1999 Asian Pacific Crossroads calendar, while working during the weekends and going to school in L.A. during the week.

"It was scary. A lot of times, I would take a leap of faith and do a lot of experimentation," Weston describes this learning process. Yet, upon accomplishing the goal, it dawned on him that he could still photograph.

Photography has always been his life and passion, his only inspiration. It had been heartbreaking for the artist to learn that he would never be able to photograph again. But the completion of the Asian Pacific Dreaming 1999 Calendar in August 1998 was proof that he could. It also opened a whole new reality for Kurt Weston, a reality which introduced him to the world of art photography, something he'd always wanted to try ever since his college years.

A feature article in the L.A. Times followed shortly in November of the same year and covered Weston's success. Not long after that, the Braille Institute invited the photographer to become part of an art show they were putting together at the Anaheim Museum of Art. They asked him to showcase some of his works. It became obvious to the artist that photography could still be part of his life, not as commercial photography, but as fine art photography.

Besides, while living with AIDS and visual loss, it would have been practically impossible for Weston to get back into commercial photography because of the amount of energy it required, but he could definitely photograph artistically. So he started devoting his attention to art photography, which later allowed him to display some of his early pieces, like The Runway, and thus further contribute to his artistic career.

Along the way, Kurt Weston realized that the imagery he created through his art was very powerful and very experimental because it was dealing with issues he had experienced personally in his day-to-day life. And, in time, as Weston's life continued to evolve and transform, so did the source of inspiration for his artwork.

It's only natural for the body of work Weston created during the eighties to be inspired by his friends' and his own experience with AIDS. Living with a terminal illness has allowed the artist to discover and connect to a more complex reality, one that resides somewhere between the physical and metaphysical spheres of human existence. Being so many times on the brink of death, Weston has become very conscious of the multidimensional world surrounding him. The physical reality was only a small part of this world. There was something more to it. The artist could only wonder if this something had anything to do with the chi energy—the energy of life pulsing with such strength through his body— the acupuncturist had mentioned at the SWAN workshops.

Or maybe it had to do with the survivors the artist had met at SWAN and from whom he learned to keep alive the belief in his ability to survive AIDS and turn it away from a sure death sentence and into something more manageable. Along the years, these survivors, Weston's "first angels," have inspired his life and also his art. Elements of the artist's view of his physical and metaphysical journey towards recovery are found in works like his Blind Vision series of self-portraits that show people the physical and emotional impact that visual loss can have on an individual.

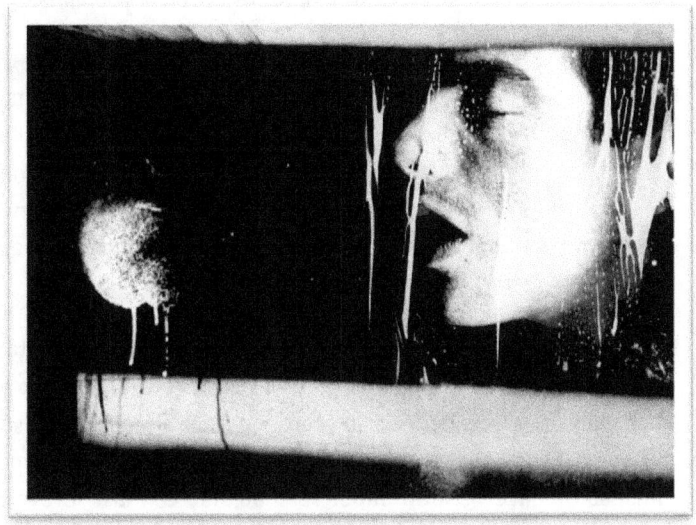

Blind Vision

The Blind Vision series is only one of Weston's works to capture an allegorical portrait of the visual artist as he traverses through his journey. In that sense, art becomes an amazing vehicle for Weston, allowing him to use his own life experiences to communicate, inspire, inform and also to visually intrigue his audience. From his perspective, Kurt Weston considers art a means through which people can experience the nature of their humanity. Art can be silly and fun, and it can be entertaining. It can communicate a tremendous amount of information, emotion, and inspiration. In today's society, consumed by superficial realities, Kurt Weston's art goes beyond the physical realm of human existence and into a metaphysical dimension, connecting with the viewer on a more profound and spiritual level.

"I think my life is meaningful," Weston comments, talking about his source of inspiration. For him life is so fragile and it can be gone in an instant. That's reason enough for the artist to capture his experience with disability, loss, pain and death in his visual art, because the experience defines him as a real person and also as an artist.

Although his most recent works include digital photography and sometimes require no camera at all (just a flat scanner which he uses to scan in people's faces and also his own face), Weston uses regular film and he prints his images on silver gelatin paper so that they can last forever. He wants future generations to be able to look at this work and say, "This was happening at this time in history and this is the impact it left on people whose lives it touched, this pandemic."

To Weston, black-and-white is a medium in itself in terms of representing reality. He doesn't want color to be an "intrusion" in his work, a "distraction" from the message his art communicates to the viewer. Black-and-white offers Weston's art a concentration of expression. And he likes that intensity, in particular in his portraits.

Kurt Weston began creating the Blind Vision series in 2000. To represent his visual disturbance described as "pieces of cotton stuck in my eye, floating every time I move my eye," the artist sprayed a glass with foaming glass cleaner and took a self-portrait sitting behind it. "You see my hand pushing away the foam, which is what I would love to do," he explains, "I would like to be able to wipe away all that cotton that keeps floating in front of my eye and get a clear view of what I want to see out in the world."

In 2003, Weston found an ad in a POZ magazine issue. The ad was calling for entries for a show about CMV retinitis. Only one entry per submission was allowed. Reading the guidelines, he told himself that the contest was made for him, so he decided to go ahead and submit. His instincts were correct—his Peering Through the Darkness, which is part of the Blind Vision series, was showcased at the Share Your Vision show at a SoHo gallery in New York City.

To go to the opening though, Weston had to pay his own trip because his artwork only won an honorable mention and the contest paid only for the prize-winning artists. Because he couldn't afford the trip, he had to "borrow and beg and steal" to make up the necessary amount. He had to look for grants that would actually be able to finance the trip. And he succeeded.

But once at the event opening, Weston became even more disappointed finding out that he was the only legally blind artist from those featured at the gallery. He was the only one walking with a cane and who actually had CMV retinitis.

There were many people who came to talk to Weston, not understanding why his entry hadn't won a prize. And listening to their opinions, the artist started to find out about what he presently refers to as "the politics of the art world," which in turn determines what's collectable art and what is not.

More than anything else, Kurt Weston had trouble understanding the politics of the disabled art world. He thought that, while dealing with the works of disabled people (like in the case of the New York City gallery), this subgroup of the art world should have had a better sense of judgment... And it bothered him that it did not.

There was yet another issue that bothered the artist. He kept wondering why disabled artists were trying so hard to cover up their disabilities instead of using their disabilities as sources of inspiration for their works. In that sense, bodies of work like Weston's Blind Vision series represent an innovative trend.

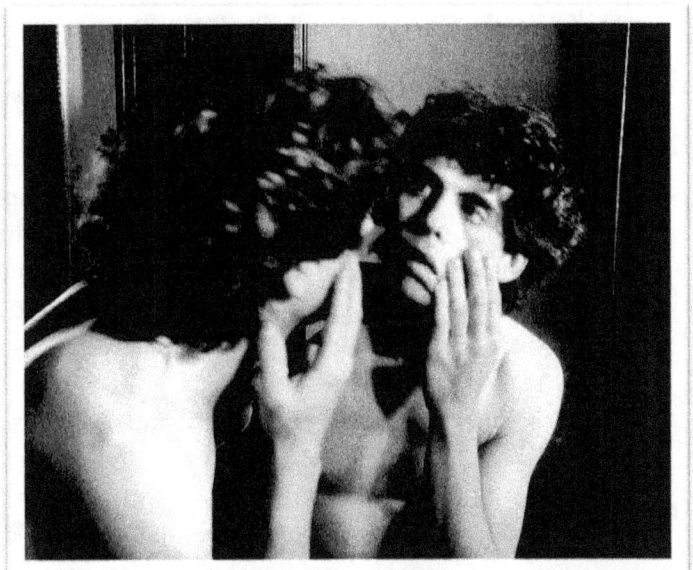

Chapter Seven: Seeing the Future

Life's Crystal Ball: Life Without Va
(Photo: Reflective Realization)

The new HAART medications have saved Kurt Weston's life. Bringing his immune system to a level that doctors considered "safe" was another story and required additional work, time, and treatments. When he initially started taking Crixivan, Kurt's immune system was virtually non-existent; therefore the medication, no matter how powerful, could not be as effective as doctors would have liked. They decided to try to boost Kurt's immune system using immunotherapy—a treatment used to rebuild an individual's impaired immune system, usually involving the administration of several cycles of immune system stimulants, called immunomodulators.

One example of an immunomodulator is Interleukin-2, a substance naturally produced by the body to stimulate its immunity. When the immune system is compromised and deteriorates below a certain level, like in the case of HIV/AIDS or cancer patients, the body cannot produce enough necessary Interleukin-2 and doctors can then intervene and administer a commercial version of the substance in order to boost the body's immunity. For AIDS patients, Interleukin-2 has the potential to halt HIV progression by maintaining the T cell count in a normal range for prolonged periods of time. Interleukin-2 can also be used for cancer treatment, to prevent the reproduction of cancerous cells.

For two consecutive years, between 1999 and 2000, Kurt Weston had to go through several Interleukin-2 cycles as part of his immunotherapy. During this time, the photographer received the medication several times a day, five days per cycle, every other month.

The treatment was helpful and definitely necessary, because the stronger Kurt's immune system was getting, the better the new HAART medications could help him regain his health and allow him to live an almost normal life. But the treatment also had severe side effects, similar to the ozone therapy ones, including a hundred and four degree fevers and rigors. And because of these side effects, by the second day on Interleukin-2, Kurt started feeling very sick. On the third day, he was holding on to dear life.

Doctors had to prescribe several medications to control the side effects and help him complete the treatment cycles. Kurt ended up taking Demoral, a powerful pain medication that knocked him out, and also various over the counter pain killers, like aspirin, for the rigors. After each Interleukin-2 cycle Kurt was going through several days of convalescence before he could start feeling better and getting on with his life again, only to resume his therapy a mere month later.

Kurt Weston survived the treatment and, two years later, he completed all the required immunotherapy cycles. As a result, his immune system eventually started to get better and his T cell count soared from three to six hundred seventy. CMV was again inactive in his body, yet the damage the virus had caused in his eyes was permanent.

To this day, in order to maintain whatever sight he has left, the photographer has to put daily prednisone drops in his eyes. The drops burn his eyes but allow him to continue photographing and creating visual art.

Previously, the disease had forced Kurt to reduce his life to bare survival. The new antiretroviral medications—the HAART regimens—started giving back not only his health, but also the chance to live his life once again, more fully. So, shortly after his graduation from the Institute for Junior Blind, Kurt started going out again using the ACCESS public transportation. He could resume attending the Positive

Friends meetings and get back in touch with individuals he'd originally met there.

It was during these meetings that he met Thomas Nylund, a historian with a special love for Roman Catholic history and theology. Thomas, who was several years older than Kurt, had AIDS and hepatitis. He continued teaching history until he got really sick and couldn't do it anymore. Thomas became an ordained priest in the American Orthodox and Catholic Church, which a lot of people did not recognize as a valid religion. But Father Thomas—as people came to know him by—always took it seriously. He had a great photographic memory and was one of those people who would give a two-hour answer to the seemingly most insignificant question he'd be asked.

In time, as they started to know each other better, Thomas started, ever so slowly, to take Va's place. He started driving Kurt everywhere the photographer needed to go and was everywhere Kurt was. The two became great buddies and even talked about renting an apartment together. They ended up living right across the street from each other.

The photographer appreciated everything Thomas was doing for him, and although Thomas would have liked to take Va's place on a more intimate level and to become Kurt's partner, the photographer, as amazed as he was by his friend's intellectual abilities, wasn't interested in taking their relationship to the next level.

By 2000, Kurt's health started to improve and he became more accustomed to getting around and more familiar with the rules imposed by his vision limitations. Yet, he still had problems seeing people and, therefore, meeting new people. In addition, because Thomas was always around, the two were always together, sometimes giving the false impression that they were a couple.

That year Kurt decided to join a workout group, which was organized by the AIDS Service Foundation (ASF) in Orange County. Because he and Thomas always arrived to the gym together, nobody in the workout group really made any serious attempts to connect with either of them.

There were many people attending the gym. Some of them were senior members, while others were newcomers. Although it was difficult for Kurt to distinguish people's faces clearly, he became aware of a particular new member who started showing up at the gym on a regular basis. Occasionally eavesdropping on the new guy's conversations with others in the gym, Kurt concluded that the man of his interest had to be a nice guy. Yet, when Kurt tried to approach him, the mystery man's face would turn beet-red and he would walk away. "He wouldn't talk to me," Kurt recalls. "He was non-conversant."

The photographer found out that his name was Terry Roberts and wished he could break the ice and talk to him, but he wasn't quite sure where that would lead because Terry kept coming to the workout group with another man, a friend of his, and Kurt didn't know if they were in a relationship or only buddies. Months later, when they started dating, Terry confessed to Kurt that because he always saw

Kurt and Thomas together, he also assumed that the two were lovers. Terry also pointed out that the workout group was not their first encounter...

At the time, Terry was on the Board of Directors of a small local AIDS support group, fighting to get some of the Ryan White funds. And for that he had to attend the HIV Planning Council meetings, the same meetings Kurt was attending in order to ask for federal funds necessary to continue the vitamin coop program he had initially started in 1996, when he was still a newcomer to Orange County and to the AIDS Service Foundation.

Although he noticed Kurt at the meetings, Terry had never tried to personally introduce himself to Kurt or to contact the photographer in any way. But it seemed that fate was giving both men a second chance.

While at the gym and despite his shyness, Terry still wanted to get to know Kurt better, but he wasn't ready to do it all by himself. So, he decided to invite the entire workout group for a Labor Day BBQ party at his house. At the time Terry had moved back in with his parents to help his mother care for his father who had Alzheimer's. So, he planned and put together the party and told his mother about Kurt, eager to hear her impression on his potential future date.

It turned out that Terry's mother liked Kurt and gave the future couple the thumbs up. Meanwhile, Kurt didn't have the slightest idea why he was invited to the party or the real reason for the party itself. After all, Kurt barely knew Terry or anybody else at the gym. In retrospect, the photographer believes that it was actually his dog who gave him a sign that Terry was, indeed, "the one" for him.

Like his master, Kurt's now aging dog is also a survivor. After Va's death, Kurt continued to stay in touch with Va's family. So, when they had a litter of puppies from their Springer Spaniel, Kurt set his heart on one of the puppies and decided it was going to be his, no matter what. Kurt even named his future pet Quasi, for Quasimodo, the protagonist's name in the 1831 Victor Hugo's novel The Hunchback of Notre Dame that tells the story of a man born with extreme deformities, who was found abandoned on the steps of Notre Dame on Quasimodo Sunday (the first Sunday after Easter)—hence his name.

Despite Kurt's dreams for his furry friend, Va's family had other plans for the litter and already had a potential buyer for Quasi. They were just waiting for the puppy to get old enough to be sold.

But Kurt never gave up. He started visiting the dog on a regular basis, bringing toys and treats, and trying to get to know Quasi better. When Va's brother, who also had chosen a puppy for himself, started stealing Quasi's toys and treats and giving them to his pup, Kurt started bringing even more goodies, so that there would be some left for his dog, too.

One day when Kurt stopped by to see Quasi, he found out that the pup had fallen into a bucket of ice-cold water and that it had been trapped there the entire night. The only way to stay alive was by holding on with its front paws to the edge of the bucket to keep its nose over the water level.

Va's family had found Quasi in the morning, paddling in the bucket, barely alive. They pulled it out of the bucket but later on it became clear that the nightlong ordeal had damaged the dog somehow because it started having seizures—would walk and fall, and then start shaking, while foam started coming out of its mouth.

Quasi's seizures went on for weeks and when it became obvious that it wasn't going to get any better, the family decided that the puppy was "damaged goods." They could never sell it anymore, so they offered it to Kurt. "If you still want it, we'll let you have it," they said.

Of course, Kurt wanted his dog. He started to prepare healthy meals for Quasi and feed it vitamins. He took his dog to the vet to get all the necessary shots and exams. And, in time, Quasi started to get better and grew more beautiful, stronger and taller than all the other dogs from the litter. "It was so amazing," Kurt says, "'cause I knew when I first set my eyes on him that he was gonna be my dog. And he ended up being my dog."

After he met Terry, Kurt invited him over to his place and offered to cook dinner for their first date. And when Terry walked in, he saw Quasi. "Ah, you have a dog," he said and then he walked right over to the couch and sat down and petted the dog.

In response, Quasi started wagging its tail, getting more and more excited. From the other side of the room, Kurt watched the scene amazed by his dog's behavior, because he had dated other people before meeting Terry, but Quasi had never responded to any of them as affectionately, if at all. The dog was usually pleasant with Kurt's previous dates, but had never shown any excitement around either of them.

But in Terry's case, Quasi stretched right over Terry's lap, almost pinning him to the couch, as if to say "You're not going anywhere!"

So Kurt interpreted his dog's behavior as a sign that they should "keep" Terry for good. Soon after they started forming a relationship, Quasi started connecting to Kurt's new partner. These days, the aging dog is more Terry's than it is Kurt's.

***

Kurt and Terry complement each other on many levels, helping each other out and being a great support to their friends. In 2002, they had to take Thomas Nylund to San Francisco to a hospital that specialized in liver transplants and post-surgery therapies, because he was in desperate need of a liver transplant.

Thomas had to wait for eight months for a transplant. While doing so, his health completely deteriorated and he started looking horribly sick. The illness and the medications he had to take caused him to lose all his fat and muscle. In time, Thomas became skin and bones, while his stomach filled with fluid that doctors needed to take out on a regular basis.

By the time the three of them made it to San Francisco, doctors took one look at Thomas and told Kurt and Terry that their friend had only a few days left to live. A liver transplant was out of the question.

Not knowing what else to do next, they took Thomas to a friend's house to spend the night. It was in that house that Kurt saw him sitting in a chair by the window and took a picture of him. Thomas died two days later.

Kurt decided to call the photograph The Last Light because his friend was seeing the light of day for the last time. He had been a big light for many people and helped the HIV/AIDS community for many long years. Father Thomas had also been a big light for the artist.

***

Before meeting Terry, the photographer used to live in a terrible HUD apartment in a really bad neighborhood. The place was unsafe. At times Kurt was afraid he was going to go back home to find the building burnt down and his expensive photography equipment destroyed, or that someone would break into his apartment and steal his things.

Kurt had serious reasons to be concerned, especially when most of the people living in that building were heroin addicts. One day, one of his neighbors got so high on drugs that he set his mattress on fire by accident. The experience started pulling the photographer back down to the bare level of surviving, and although the fears and insecurities that came with living in the HUD buildings were different from his fear of dying of AIDS during the early days of the epidemic, the effect was similar.

"Every time you go back down to just surviving," Weston explains, "you can't really go forward 'cause you only focus on getting to the next day. [Only] when you can break out of that survival mode you can move forward because you can focus [on putting] your energy into things that will allow you to move forward."

In a way, meeting his new partner jumpstarted Kurt's moving forward. After getting to know each other better, it was time for them to take the next step forward and start a more serious relationship and move in together. Terry offered to use his savings as down payment on a house. They found a nice place in a very safe neighborhood, where they both could feel comfortable. Their new home also allowed Kurt the freedom to move forward with his life and his art. He started by converting the garage into his photo studio.

It is always important for any individual to have someone around to share together the joys of life and face its obstacles. It is extremely important for somebody having to deal with visual impairment and who is also trying to accomplish something with his visual art to find someone who shares not only his dedication to living, but also to creating art. For Kurt, that important someone is Terry.

He drives Kurt to his doctor's appointments, to school and to all the events the photographer needs to attend. This offering has helped Kurt take a step closer to realizing his dreams and allowed him the safe haven of a place where he feels free to create and work towards his ideals, a place where he doesn't have to struggle to survive from one day to the next, but only to focus on his goals.

Kurt and Terry complement each other in many ways. Kurt helps his partner by focusing on his wellbeing. For instance, when they first started dating, Kurt realized that Terry wasn't taking any nutritional supplements and that his medications weren't helping much at all either. While Terry believed that he could deal with the side effects and continue treatment the way it was, Kurt wasn't too convinced that it was the best idea. Besides, he didn't want to see his partner, his "soul mate," suffer when he didn't have to.

So, he used his power of persuasion to get Terry to start taking vitamins and therapeutic nutrients. Kurt also helped him change to a better drug regimen and also to a better physician. It wasn't long until he started scheduling their doctor's appointments at the same time, so that they could both go together.

Terry might be Kurt's eyes on the way to the doctor, but in the examination room, Kurt becomes his partner's voice, because Terry is not the kind of person who would tell doctors about everything that's bothering him. So, even to this day, every time Terry refuses to talk about what's bothering him and tries to paint a pretty picture that everything is just fine with him, Kurt jumps in to inform their physician of his partner's full list of aches and pains, of meds that work and especially those that don't.

Kurt's updates are a reality check that usually gets the doctor to start asking questions, thus forcing Terry to answer them. And if he refuses, Kurt answers the questions for him, and he's more than willing to do it, to make sure that his soul mate stays healthy. He believes that, otherwise, Terry's health would get worse. And Kurt is not willing to let important issues like his partner's health to slip away.

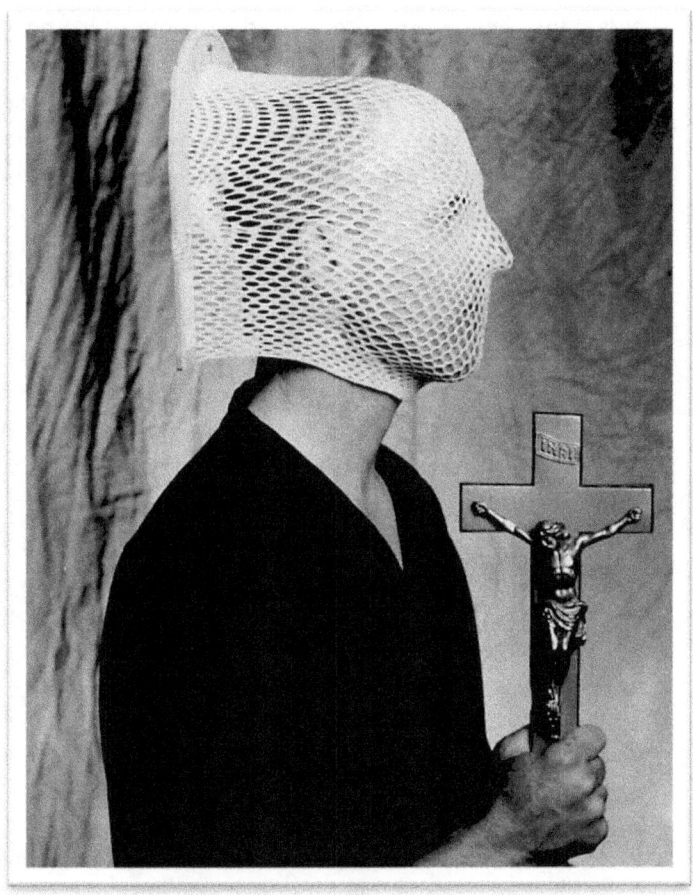

Chapter Eight: Modern Crucifixion
Warrior Within: A Source of Strength

In 2000, Kurt's younger brother was diagnosed with
T cell lymphoma. Starting with a cancerous tumor behind his

heart, the metastases spread throughout his body, threatening to take his life. To win his battle with cancer, Kurt's brother had to undergo two years of chemotherapy and radiation. Because the treatment involved radiating parts of his head, doctors had to apply a mask over his face and head to shelter his brain from being radiated.

Throughout the entire ordeal, Kurt stood by his brother's side, accompanying him to his doctor's appointments and participating in discussions regarding best suitable, available treatments and therapies. His brother won his battle with cancer, partly because he was inspired by Kurt's dedication to survive AIDS. "If Kurt can survive, I can do it, too," he declared. The mask he had to wear during his radiation sessions also inspired the photographer's Modern Crucifixion, in which his brother appears wearing a mask over his head and holding a crucifix in his hands.

The crucifix signifies the suffering and pain of the Christ. In modern society, it may signify the suffering and pain of people living with life threatening diseases, like cancer or HIV/AIDS.

One cannot talk about crucifixion without getting into the whole issue of stigmata—the holes through which the nails permeated Christ's hands and feet. Modern stigmata marks can be of a physical, cultural or lifestyle matter. In a contemporary society, with a deep foundation in computer-generated "beauty" and man-made "perfection," living with a physical disability is many times considered below the acceptable "norm," and, in turn, can attract unwanted attention, which can further lead to stigma. Those who fit in this particular category can become victims of modern stigmatization.

Handicaps—that is losing the ability to use part of one's body—and also disease can lead to such stigma. Cancer, for example, may require severe chemotherapies or surgeries, may cause one's hair loss or changes in physical appearance; therefore flagging the individual as having—or having had—cancer and, sometimes bringing unwanted attention or behaviors towards a cancer patient. But, while people may also react to a cancer diagnosis with a feeling of pity, sorrow or even fear, many times their reaction is completely different when it comes to so-called "shameful" diseases, as HIV/AIDS is sometimes still considered.

Maybe the most society-stigmatized disease ever is AIDS. The reason for the HIV/AIDS prejudice has changed over the last quarter century or more, as it did the face of AIDS itself, which refers, really, to the whole physical appearance associated with HIV/AIDS patients and which, today, mimics the side effects to the newest medications and treatments.

The modern-day face of AIDS is not a face of death anymore, but rather is defined by new terms like "Crixi (or Crix) bellies," "PI pouches," "buffalo humps" or "sunken cheeks [syndromes]." It is partly a face of HAART regimens, the very medications vital for patients to sustain a normal life and lifespan. Therefore, especially in North America and Western Europe, the contemporary face of AIDS is associated with physical deformations that sometimes can transform a patient's appearance beyond recognition.

Due to the new protease inhibitors he was on, called d4T, Kurt Weston was also starting to grow a buffalo hump and a stomach pouch (also known as a P.I. pouch). When he asked his doctor to switch him to a drug that wouldn't distort his body, his doctor told him about a new medication at the time, an entry inhibitor that was coming up the pipeline and becoming available.

In 2003, FDA approved a medication called Fuzeon (or T20) supposed to fight HIV by not allowing the virus to enter the T cell. Because it is difficult to manufacture, the drug is extremely expensive and available only as an injection. Studies have shown that AIDS patients who are on Fuzeon may get skin rashes where they self-administer the shots, or some may become more prone to developing pneumonia.

Doctors put the photographer on Fuzeon and a combination of other medications. While on Fuzeon (taken in combination with other antiretroviral medications), Kurt has experienced very few side effects and he liked that very much. Also, to make best use of the medication and his time, he had no choice but to quickly learn how to integrate his shots into his daily schedule.

Ever since his diagnosis, AIDS has been a constant variable in the equation that describes Kurt Weston's existence. In time and with the appearance of new treatments, the threat of his disease has turned from immediate to manageable. These days, AIDS has become more of a constant companion in his life rather than a threat, but it continues to influence, at least partly, all decisions, minor and major alike, that he has to make—be they related to his studies, to traveling or eating his meals.

In general, some medications have to be taken with food, while others before or after meals at precise times each day, several times throughout the day, for the rest of the AIDS patient's life. For this reason, people living with the virus and on such medications always have to take their treatments into consideration when planning their daily activities.

On mornings when he had to make it to school early, Kurt made sure to get all his medications ready the previous night before going to sleep. He lined up all his pills so they would be ready for him to grab on his way out the door the following morning.

But pills are only a small part of Kurt's treatment. He also has to give himself daily injections.

To be able to self-administer the Fuzeon, he first has to prepare the fluid—that is to put sterile water in the Fuzeon vial and get it hydrated. Then he would store the container in the refrigerator until he's ready to use it, which should be within twenty-four hours. The daily two Fuzeon shots have minimum side effects on Kurt, but, on the other hand, they're also "a pain in the ass," as he calls them, because they require a lot of knowledge, work, patience, and time. And Kurt has to deal with these treatments and medications every single day, no matter how busy or fast pace his day may be.

For a while, Kurt was also taking a trial medication supposed to reduce his lipodystrophy (or body fat mal-distribution), which is a side effect to some HAART regimens. This was a new and experimental drug supposed to keep his fat from accumulating in all the wrong places. Therefore, every single day, after getting his first medication started, he had to take his first dose of pills, and then start hydrating his second, trial medication. Kurt had to self-administer two vials of this medication, daily, in order to see any results. For a while it seemed to work nicely and he started losing his P.I. belly. He also learned to wear clothes that would hide whatever was left of it… Eventually, Kurt had to stop taking the trial medication because of its various side effects.

Medication also interferes with patients' traveling schedules. Kurt Weston avoids being away from home for longer than a week, partly because he doesn't have enough room in his suitcase to carry medication for more than six or seven days at a time. When he travels, the photographer has to bring with him the Fuzeon kits containing the syringes, alcohol swabs, medications, sterile water and all the vials with the actual medication. He has to pack them so that they don't break or get damaged in any way, and then pray to God that at the airport nobody stops him to ask why he's carrying all those syringes and vials with him.

The entire process is a hassle, but Weston prefers it to taking lots of pills that give him lots of negative and powerful side effects. With the Fuzeon injections, he only experiences a hard tiny bump at the place where he administers the injection, and only because it takes awhile for the drug to disperse from under his skin. But to take a drug whose only problem is that it has to be injected is not a big deal for Weston. He has been on other drugs that gave him all kinds of "unpleasant" side effects.

Some of the medications he's tried throughout his years of living with AIDS gave him neuropathy (which is numbness in his extremities, hands and feet), while others caused him to have severe diarrhea, "Like I take the drug and an hour later I'm having bowel movements, five minutes apart," he recalls. Yet other drugs had the power to send him into a complete druggy and groggy state of being.

Weston considers Sustiva a "horrible drug" that used to send him into a perpetual delusion. While struggling to minimize the side effects as much as possible, he first tried taking the medication at night, before going to sleep. But as it turned out, while the pills were making him dizzy, they were also keeping him from falling asleep. Not willing to give up, he then tried taking Sustiva during the afternoon, several hours before going to bed, but that made him feel "out of it," as if he were on sleeping pills for the rest of the day.

Norvir, a protease inhibitor that came in oversize pills, gave him diarrhea, and because it had a lot of alcohol in it, it also made him sleepy. He had to take eight capsules of the medication in the morning and another eight at nighttime, daily.

Drugs like Zerit and ddI gave him neuropathy. While he hasn't been on these medications in quite a long time, the numbness in his extremities has started to improve slowly, yet it has never gone away completely. When it comes to neuropathy, the photographer still has his good days and his bad days, especially when he has to stand or walk for a long time. Even these days, he still experiences a tingling sensation in his limbs, although it's not a constant pain anymore.

Other side effects can be even more serious, depending on the type of medications the patients are on. The new HAART regimens have radically transformed the progression and manifestation of AIDS, but their unquestionable benefits came with a price tag. While the unattractive fat accumulations caused by these drugs cannot always be noticed, it doesn't mean that they cannot cause significant problems for patients. Sometimes the erratic fat accumulations happen deep inside the body, in the arteries, causing AIDS patients high cholesterol and triglycerides levels, thus increasing the risk of blocking their arteries, which can lead to heart attacks or even death.

Some AIDS patients on certain HAART regimens require open-heart surgery. Weston has never had to go through anything like that, but a good friend of his who was on the new drug regimens wasn't that lucky. She died of a massive coronary. She was forty-eight.

Same meds supposed to keep HIV from replicating in patients' bodies can also be responsible for the new look of the perpetually changing "face of AIDS," sketched by the fat accumulations anomalies associated with the new HAART regimens. The dents and valleys of fat deposits redefine patients' entire physical appearance, transforming individuals into "human freaks" because their stomachs are blown out like balloons, while everything else is shrinking away and veins are sticking out on their arms and legs, and they look like someone starving in Africa.

Sometimes their disfiguration is so advanced, so severe, that patients refuse to go out in public, because they can cover everything else but their faces. The loss of fat in their faces gives them a gnawed appearance, which can be quite drastic. As a result, many of them find no other solution but to become prisoners in their own homes, of their own disease, this time not because of KS lesions, but of the very medications that have radically turned their lives around.

Some patients are even willing to risk their physical lives in order to be able to have some kind of social life, because, after all, what good is feeling healthy when they cannot enjoy life. So, they decide to stop taking their AIDS medications and go on so-called "drug holidays" until they start regaining some of their normal physical appearance.

Some others ask professionals to inject substances like Newfill in their faces to regain at least part of their normal looks. The treatment is very expensive and costs thousands of dollars for one session. Most of the time, it is not covered by medical insurance. In addition, the patients need to go through several sessions in order for them to see any improvements.

In 2006, the Food and Drug Administration has announced the approval of a new once-a-day pill for treating HIV/AIDS. The pill, called Atripla, became available in the

United States and it was supposed to be made available to fifteen other countries, including South Africa, Uganda, Botswana, Rwanda, Haiti, and Vietnam.

The FDA approval of Atripla offers a potentially easier way for HIV/AIDS patients to keep up with their medications, thus allowing them more time to concentrate on other aspects of their lives. For patients who cannot or don't want to deal with the drug side effects two or three times a day, a once-a-day pill can have its benefits, but that doesn't mean that it works for all patients.

Confirmed by the early 2007 HIV/AIDS updates, medical professionals consider Atripla a convenient once a day pill. It is not a breakthrough and not a one-pill-fits-all HIV patients. Many newly diagnosed individuals and those co-infected with hepatitis cannot take Atripla. It can take one to three months or more to adjust to the medication. Some patients develop rashes severe enough to switch to other regimens. There are no studies yet showing that Atripla is safer, less toxic or more capable to increase lifespan than other medications. Related post-exposure prophylaxis studies are expensive because they require a large sample size.

Typically, there has to be a certain level of medications in a patient's body in order to keep the virus in check. So, taking one large pill a day, at the beginning of the day, creates a significant stress on the liver, because the liver is the organ through which all drugs are processed. A once-a-day pill may be convenient to the patient, but it may not be as convenient to the body that has to process a huge dose of medications and then sustain itself throughout the day. In addition, the one-time-a-day medication is not really a new drug, but rather the combination of three drugs already available on the market.

"[Basically, pharmaceutical companies] are taking these three drugs and putting them together in one pill," Weston comments, "and they probably up the amount of drug in those pills, because it has to get you through twenty-four hours in one dose. So, you're probably taking the drugs that are currently available already, but you're just taking them in one combination pill."

Kurt Weston is not impressed by the once-a-day treatment because he doesn't really like the idea of taking "one large blasting dose" of medication once a day. Therefore, although his doctor offered him the option to put him on a once-a-day medication, he rejected the idea and opted for continuing with his twice or three times a day treatment.

The photographer is more interested in phasing out his drug therapy, keeping the drugs at a plateau level and doing it in a way that would not stress his organs. To him, learning how to deal with his medication begins with learning to understand his entire body, his entire universe—the physical and spiritual part of it—something he learned to master while in Chicago, through his SWAN experience and the first "warriors" he met at Test Positive Aware.

While doing so, Weston believes that his surviving AIDS has helped him resurrect not only as a person, but also as an artist. Despite all the obstacles, his AIDS and his blindness have offered him a second chance to life in general, and to his professional life, in particular. So, he took his chances and did the best he possibly could with them, while never thinking of giving up.

"Even when I was living in Chicago and I had the KS lesions, I never really wanted to just give up. I think part of it was the fear of dying," Kurt Weston confesses. "[But] I didn't just wait for it to happen. I thought, this is like a battle and I need to be a warrior. I need to go and I need to face this terror in my life head on, I can't just sit back and let this terror consume me, [but] fight and be aware of everything or anything that's out there in the world that can possibly help me fight the virus destroying me."

That was the reason behind Weston's starting the SWAN group, knowing that there were other people like him who weren't willing to give up, who wanted to survive and fight their AIDS and who were looking for any ways possible to stay alive. They were the warriors who were not just waiting to die, but rather actively trying to slow down the progress of their AIDS, be that by either experimenting with an alternative therapy, or by taking a yoga class or an acupuncture class, or trying massage therapy or meditation, or taking herbs, vitamins and therapeutic nutrients.

In that sense, organizations like Test Positive Aware or Kurt's SWAN workshops were sources of inspiration and information. They were rays of hope for attendees, pulling them through incredibly tough times when they were literally on the brink of dying. These AIDS service organizations offered people like Kurt the opportunity to actively do something about their disease, sometimes through informational seminars, workshops and other avenues through which patients could learn something about their disease and to spread the word further along to other patients. And through it all, Weston has become a source of inspiration for many others whose lives he has touched.

Over the years, the AIDS demographic has started to change. More and more women, people of color, the elderly and the youth have started getting infected at an increasing rate, and, therefore, started attending AIDS workshops and becoming involved with AIDS service organizations. As a result, the topics and focus of AIDS workshops and organizations have also started to change in order to incorporate the needs of their newest members.

***

While attending Test Positive Aware in Chicago, Kurt offered his share of comfort to people suffering and dying from the same disease that was threatening his own life. There were specific instances when he would have to call the hospital or go and visit people who were in the hospital. There were moments when he had to try to talk to patients' doctors and negotiate treatments in their name, because they were too sick to do it by themselves anymore.

Hospital visits were especially difficult before the advent of HAART regimens because there were so many people dying of AIDS. Kurt has experienced a lot of various end stages of AIDS, watching people die because there was nothing anybody could do at the time to save their lives. And all that he could do for the suffering was to be there for them and comfort them and tell them "hey, you did well." But it was frustrating and painful, because, while witnessing so much death, Kurt was himself very sick. He knew that every time he went to the hospital to witness somebody's death or dying process, it could be only days until he'd be in the same stage, dying in a hospital bed. Yet, he continued to comfort the dying, while forcing the thought of his own death to the back of his mind, all the while remaining very much aware of the possibility of his own death.

Every time Weston had to visit someone in the hospital, his stomach would go into knots, but he volunteered to do it anyway, despite the one hundred and two degree fever, the KS lesions on his face and the IV drip in his arm. That was the way he went to visit patients who were hospitalized for various reasons, yet who were all dying of AIDS.

Once he had to visit one of his friends who had cryptosporidium infection. Crypto, or cryptosporidiosis, is one of the parasitic infections common in people living with HIV. Crypto is caused by an intestinal parasite usually found in animals. People can get infected through contaminated food or public water. The parasite grows in the intestines and bile ducts and causes severe, chronic watery diarrhea with up to twenty-five bowel movements per day.

When crypto causes illness in otherwise healthy individuals, the infection goes away in one to two weeks. In people with AIDS, the infection is usually chronic.

In the case of Kurt's friend, doctors had tried treating him with antibiotics, but the infection really didn't get any better because of the patient's weakened immune system. The crypto was affecting his life so severely that, if he had to eat something, he'd immediately have massive diarrhea. He couldn't keep any food in his body. His situation was so severe that the medical professionals had to set up a portable potty next to his bed.

As Kurt sat by his bedside talking to him, his friend got up and said, "excuse me," and then he got out of the bed and set right on his potty. "... And he started shitting right in front of me because he couldn't control it," the photographer recalls. And that's how his friend had been living for a full year. He died, two weeks after that visit.

The photographer also had a friend who had AIDS and would always say that he wished he'd die before everybody else because he was afraid he was going to outlive everybody and there would be no one left to care for him when his turn would come. That seemed ridiculous to Kurt because nobody knew what could happen in time. Besides, no matter the belief, ultimately, death is a lonely process. People don't die with somebody. When they die, they do it alone. "I didn't want to think about what it's gonna be like when I'm dying," Kurt comments. "My perspective was 'I don't want to die.' Yes, it's not easy living like this, but I kept believing that somehow, somewhere, I was going to survive this and I had to keep believing and I did whatever I could to keep that hope alive."

Kurt Weston used part of that hope to run his SWAN group. The information that SWAN participants were sharing with everybody else has helped the photographer and all the other SWAN members to find and hold on to hope, because SWAN was proving to them that, indeed, there was something they could try and do in order to survive.

Sometimes the beautiful people with not a scar of AIDS on them would die first, taking the artist completely by surprise. One of these beautiful people was a stunning guy who was attending the SWAN workshops. Kurt thought that he would outlive him by a long time. As it turned out, the man had some kind of fungal infection in his lungs. He tried everything, but nothing really worked... and Kurt's prediction turned out to be wrong.

Another person the photographer thought was looking too fabulous to have AIDS was the volunteer instructor teaching yoga classes at Test Positive Aware. Kurt remembers him as an attractive man, very muscular and good-looking, someone who would obviously have lots of admirers. He was using his body to show his students all kinds of contorted positions and Kurt was always amazed at what he could do.

One day, the gorgeous instructor told his class that he had KS lesions. The news shocked everybody, Kurt in particular. But then, the yoga instructor lifted his shirt to expose the purple spots on his stomach. A few months later he stopped coming to the class.

Not long afterwards, Kurt heard that the instructor had been hospitalized and that the KS had attacked his lungs and he had problems breathing. He also had asked for Kurt to stop by and visit him and try to negotiate with his doctors about his treatment.

At the time, Kurt had already learned that ganciclovir or foscarnet, which were used to treat CMV, seemed also helpful for treating KS lesions. But when he shared what he'd learnt with the instructor's doctors, they didn't really want to talk to him and continued giving their patient chemotherapy, which depleted his immune system even more.

The volunteers who taught classes at TPA inspired Kurt to start a vitamin coop, which could provide therapeutic nutrients to people living with HIV/AIDS at a low wholesale price. Nutrients and vitamins were usually expensive, and Kurt and other people attending SWAN could not afford them, being on disability.

Later on, after moving to California, Kurt decided to continue in the tradition of SWAN and started a similar therapeutic nutrients program in Orange County at the AIDS Services Foundation, which is a local organization that services people with HIV/AIDS. But, before actually starting the program, Kurt began to talk to members of ASF and realized that many people could not afford to purchase the vitamins and nutrients even below wholesale prices. That's when he realized he needed some of the Ryan White money to make the program possible.

Named after Ryan White, the hemophiliac teenager from Indiana infected with HIV whose fight against AIDS stigma and prejudice has made the headlines, the Ryan White Comprehensive AIDS Relief Emergency (or C.A.R.E.) Act was actually signed by the Congress in 1990, and is still the nation's largest source of government funding for the uninsured and low-income people living with HIV/AIDS.

To start a nutrient therapeutic program in Orange County, Kurt had to actually join the HIV Planning Council, which is "the political eye" that decides how the Ryan White money coming from the federal government is spent. It was at one of these meetings that the photographer first met Terry.

At these meetings Kurt had to slowly and patiently explain why it was so important for people living with HIV/AIDS to take their nutrients. Kurt needed to start developing a program and he chose AIDS Service Foundation as the agency to host his nutrient program, which would end up having two parts: Vitamart, offering nutrients at half price to people living with HIV/AIDS; and Nutritional Educational Therapy (or NET), offering free nutrients to people who could not afford them.

The executive director of ASF was extremely appreciative of how Kurt's program could help people with HIV attending AIDS Service Foundation and she supported

Kurt's initiative; therefore, the Vitamart part of the program didn't take too long to start, in 1996.

But then, when Kurt began going to halfway houses to talk about the benefits of therapeutic nutrients, people with HIV/AIDS living in these places told him that there was no way they could pay for such supplements. While it was clear to him that the Vitamart program could not work for these patients, Kurt sought advice from a friend who was in the HIV Planning Council and who told the photographer to go to the Council meetings and ask for Ryan White money. But the fund was hard to get approved, especially because there were a lot of people in the Council who did not believe in therapeutic nutrients at all, saying that the whole thing was just bogus and they shouldn't spend their money on it. Therefore, the second half of the program, called Nutritional Educational Therapy, didn't happen overnight.

It wasn't until later on in 1996 that the Planning Council actually approved the money, which, in turned, allowed Kurt to get started with his NET program in 1997. To become eligible for NET, all that was necessary for patients was a prescription from their doctor and proof that their incomes were under a certain limit. It turned out that out of the fifteen hundred clients at the AIDS Service Foundation in Orange County, about three hundred fifty ended up using these nutrients, which, in turn, were available with the help of Ryan White money.

Over time, the rate of HIV infections in Orange County has gone down significantly, also partly because of people like Weston and their efforts. The accomplishment pushed the county down on the list of priorities when it came to receiving necessary HIV/AIDS-related funds. Therefore, when, as a result of the 2005 reauthorization of the Ryan White money, some funds had to be reallocated, organizations like AIDS Service Foundation in Orange County have been left to do with less money.

Throughout the years there have been many people who have tried to get rid of Weston's therapeutic nutrients program because they did not believe in it. Yet, somehow, the photographer has managed to pull it through each year and obtain the necessary funds. After 2005 though, many projects sponsored by federal funding have been annihilated, leaving Weston and others like him with not much ability to get some of the year's Ryan White money. The Orange County HIV Planning Council has announced its views on discontinuing the nutrients program in 2006. There was nothing that Weston could do to stop its annihilation and, together with it, the annihilation of other useful and successful ASF programs.

Nevertheless, there is obvious statistical evidence that nutrients and vitamins do help. Examples include studies done in several African countries.

For a long time, the South African government was against the use of antiretroviral (ARV) medications, sharing the dissident opinion that "HIV does not cause AIDS," hence the South African AIDS denialism theory that has been studied and talked about in many books and by many experts on both sides of the debate. In Africa, AIDS is sometimes thought to be part of a white-borne racist agenda, propagated by stigmatizing conceptions of African sexuality and Africa as the "origin" of AIDS. Lately, especially after the 2006 International AIDS Conference in Toronto, members of South African Treatment Action Campaign, or TAC, have advocated for the use of antiretroviral medications and for the replacement of the country's Health Minister, who was denying the medications to the general public, the theory behind it being that, if HIV doesn't cause AIDS, then the anti-HIV medications are useless.

There were studies following the progression of AIDS in a person who was not taking ARV medication. Monitoring the evolution of the disease in people who were taking nutrients and vitamins versus those who were not, these studies showed that individuals who received only the nutrients did much better than those who did not receive any nutritional therapy. Present studies show that vitamins and nutrients are also helpful for AIDS patients who are on HAART regimens.

Running the vitamin coops (in Chicago and also later on, in Orange County, was a big deal for Kurt, because he had to do everything by himself. He had to take the orders, collect the money, send in the orders, get the supplements delivered, unpack them and put them in the right bags for those who came to pick them up or call the people to tell them that their supplements arrived, and to verify that their supplements were delivered.

It was a lot of work, but the result helped people not only physically, but also mentally. Part of it was because people who were deciding to take the nutrients were actually deciding to do something about their AIDS and to take control of their lives. By taking those nutrients, they were actively doing something positive for their ability to survive. Therefore, the vitamin coop wasn't only about selling and buying nutrients, or swallowing a pill, but it also had an emotional and psychological element attached to it, an element also found in programs like SWAN that helped people survive and, in the process, become warriors at battle with their virus.

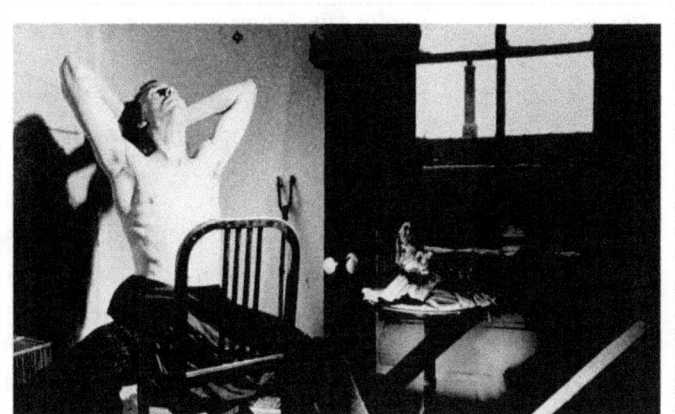

Chapter Nine: Arrival of the Angel

Message from a Warrior

Although they may not be aware of a time without AIDS, today's youth also cannot remember the early years of the epidemic, simply because many of them were not around some thirty years ago. Some of those who were, though, have chosen to remain indifferent to the epidemic, simply because AIDS has never affected them or someone they cared about. Simply put, because AIDS has never been in their backyard.

It is impossible for some individuals to truly relate to someone else's loss unless they experience loss themselves. It is difficult to understand the true depth of human suffering for those who've never lived through any kind of disaster or life-altering situation. It is almost normal to feel disconnected from someone else's tragedy unless, somehow, that tragedy hits home. This idea holds true when it comes to the "AIDS problem" that doesn't seem to go away, and also to the Iraq war—it just doesn't mean anything to many of those not fighting in the war, who don't know how things really are on the frontline.

Kurt Weston knows too well the feeling of loss, fear and isolation usually associated with such extreme situations. He can relate to soldiers in a war because, like them, he has been fighting his own war with a deadly disease. Just like the soldiers on the battlefield, he has experienced the AIDS battlefield where he has witnessed death and looked it in the eye, while trying to comfort those who were losing their own war with AIDS, those who were beyond any medical help, who were suffering and dying in front of him.

The photographer has also experienced the feeling of overwhelming hopelessness associated with the beginning of the epidemic, when visiting his friends in the hospital two or three times a week, watching as a disfiguring and grotesque disease was slowly killing them, while there was nothing that anybody could do to save them.

Today there is virtually no country in the world that is free of HIV/AIDS, but the evolution of the disease and treatment progress vary from one country to another. AIDS is still a death sentence for many people in Africa, sometimes simply because they don't have the appropriate medications. Yet, because their suffering happens continents away, it doesn't mean much for many people living in Western countries. This is only one aspect of the indifference and denial with which many individuals who live in today's American society, for instance, treat real-life issues happening in the world.

It is sad that too many people live nowadays as if "in a mental insanity," where reality and illusion overlap and become something unidentifiable. "If you look at it," Kurt Weston says, "our whole society is permeated with illusion."

Indeed, it's much more convenient to live in a world of illusions, a "happy-bubble" offering individuals a deceptive sense of security and comfort and an askew perspective of the world outside the "happy bubble," filtered by the various version of perfection, material richness and beauty on the covers of glossy magazines and TV screens. Each day people spend long hours watching a tube or a screen and being awed by the glitz and glory of a Hollywood world they know nothing about, but only think they do. While the images streaming in front of their eyes start shaping their perspective of the world beyond their TV tube or screen, their minds refuse—and later become unable—to deal with what's waiting for them in the real world.   The TV is usually a distraction from the harsh reality of life, rather than a tool through which people can get educated and informed in order to better understand and deal with the real world.

Sometimes it is hard to live beyond illusions. It is difficult to recognize what's real and learn to deal with it, because most of the time reality is pain and only sometimes glory. But at least reality is not fakery.

The truth is that there is more bad in the world than there is good, that too many wars have started in the name of religion and religious beliefs, and that there are some religious leaders so extraordinarily powerful that they manipulate their followers to believe that blowing themselves up in order to take along with them innocent lives is what their god asks of them. The truth is that, eventually, everybody is going to die; that, at some point, every person is going to get sick or old and then realize that it's not easy living as an elderly person or with a disease. "It's hard to live in the reality all the time," Weston says, "but would you rather live [in it] with your eyes open or with [them] closed?"

People have to make decisions every day of their lives. When they are forced into extreme situations like a terminal disease, or a natural or man-made calamity, making these decisions becomes even more complicated and presents individuals with issues they don't really want to deal with. As a result, issues like mortality and basic survival become more real, almost tangible.

In the case of AIDS, many of those infected during the beginning of the epidemic decided that it wasn't worth it to put up a fight, maybe because they thought they didn't have a chance to win the battle against the disease to begin with. Therefore, they took a few sleeping pills and ended their suffering.

Others, like Kurt Weston, decided to try to survive AIDS and deal with the pain associated with the disease. The photographer has stayed by his decision even when he was very much aware of an easier way out.

This attitude has served as a starting point in his life after being diagnosed with AIDS, because in order to fight the battle with the disease, he had first to accept it as a permanent part of his life. Years later the same happened with his accepting the permanent loss of his sight. Accepting loss as part of reality is no simple thing, especially when what is lost forever used to be an intrinsic part of an individual's life. For Weston, a photographer, an artist who could paint with light, the loss of his ability to perceive light was devastating. But even this loss could not stop him from being a photographer, quite the contrary.

Throughout his life, Kurt Weston has never mistaken life for an illusion. Being diagnosed and having to live with the disease, he realized that he had to accept the fact that he could not escape his AIDS—and, after that, the related visual loss. To this day, he wakes up every morning having to deal twenty-four hours a day with his own modern crucifixion and to accept his own reality, in order to be able to make the best of it. And he is not alone in his struggle.

Other people have to deal with their own realities, experiencing their own modern crucifixions and carrying their own crosses. Some may have to deal with the realization that they have cancer, or that they've been in a terrible accident or war, which left them impaired for the rest of their lives, or that there are bombs going over their heads that force them to live in constant fear and terror. And still, they wake up each day to face their realities and deal with them the best they possibly can.

"The reality is that life is pain," Kurt Weston comments. "There are little bits of joy and happiness, but ultimately there's pain, and there's suffering and sorrow and issues of all kinds. And once people realize that that's basically what life is really about, only then they can get on with it instead of just living in a fake fantasy world of glitz and glamour, instead of just living in denial."

During his Positively Speaking workshops, Weston would talk to students in schools across Orange County about the reality of life and of AIDS as part of life. It would always surprise the photographer that most students would not realize that AIDS can leave people blind; that students are shocked to find out that living with AIDS is much more complicated than just swallowing a few pills or that the medications he has to take every day to stay alive cost him up to eighty thousand dollars a year, or that AIDS can violate patients' health and wellbeing but also wipe out their bank accounts; that that patients become eligible for public assistance only after their savings are completely depleted.

"It's strange that people are ignorant about how they [might] get AIDS," Kurt Weston comments. "We need a lot more of [education and prevention, but] unfortunately [too often the focus is still placed solely on] abstinence. It would be nice if young people could abstain from sexual behavior, but that's not the reality. The reality is that a young person with hormones coursing through the body is going to engage in sexual behavior. And it's to [these] individuals that we need to provide safer sex messages in terms of how to do it safely and prevent getting infected."

***

As it happens with everything in life, there are always two sides to a story. It's part of the duality that governs our entire existence. The same stands true in the world of AIDS, forcing individuals to walk a very fine line in order to keep focused on what's really important.

One aspect of the duality of AIDS may be explained by the very life-saving medications introduced in the mid-nineties. The HAART regimens had a so-called "Lazarus effect," the coming back to life from the brink of death effect on HIV/AIDS patients. Before the advent of the new antiretroviral medications, AIDS was a feared disease that sentenced its victims to an agonizing and silent dying process. Back then, too many of Weston's friends got sick and died horrible deaths. Back then, infected people had to deal with the reality that they were HIV positive and there was nothing that they could do to help themselves. The photographer can still recall the emotional and psychological stress his friends had to bear dealing with their disease, its discrimination, and stigma.

In the mid-nineties, as a direct result of HAART regimens, people living with HIV/AIDS started to get back some of the normality of their lives. Because of the new medications, it didn't take them long to start feeling well enough to resume their work. They were not "damaged goods" anymore. Rather, they could once again consider themselves successful members of society. For them, AIDS did not equal DEATH anymore. They were not dying of the disease anymore and they refused to be treated as if they were; therefore, they wanted to end the stigma and the "AIDS is a death sentence" mind-set.

But the mind-set didn't quite go away so fast. Companies were not hiring people who, they believed, didn't have much longer to live. And so, AIDS patients started to conceal their disease. They could do it because they were healthy enough and had enough energy again. Unfortunately, not long into their new treatments, patients also started experiencing new side effects and, with them, the new face of AIDS, which soon could be easily identified. And so, the AIDS-related stigma and prejudice couldn't quite go away either.

"People [ask] me 'why are you trying to get your MFA or working so hard on your career, why don't you enjoy the time you have left?'" Weston says, remembering the remarks from when he was working on his MFA in photography. "I don't see myself as a person who's gonna die anytime soon and I want to do something with my life... You know how horrific it would be for someone to tell me that 'I'm not gonna give you a grant to go back to school because you're basically a dead person'?"

When the HAART regimens were made available, and then, in time, started saving and extending lives, the new treatments slowly began to transform AIDS from a terminal illness to a manageable one. With the occasional exceptions, in Western countries AIDS does not equal SILENCE anymore, nor does it equal DEATH, unless people let it. Therefore, nowadays, some relate living with HIV/AIDS to endurance; to the responsibility of keeping up with daily life-long treatments and dealing with their side effects; to the ability of juggling a variety of issues of a wide range of intensities on a daily basis, while still being able to sustain a high level of normality in life; or to learning the art of living fully, while being infected with a still-deadly virus.

Yet, sometimes, the very idea of people "living" with HIV/AIDS and not "dying" of it anymore translates into the illusion that AIDS is somehow not a problem anymore. As a result, complacency starts settling in because AIDS is not considered an immediate life-threatening disease anymore.

The non-imminent deadly danger associated with the disease also means less funds being allocated to AIDS support groups. Therefore, non-profits in need of these funds have to find new ways of keeping people interested in the disease and its cause. As a result, there are a lot of mixed messages going out regarding HIV/AIDS, affecting mostly the young generation that has never lived in a time when AIDS was a sure death sentence, and, therefore, cannot understand the magnitude of such a disease.

Most of those who are not infected do not have a clue what it means and what it takes to live with the virus. Several years ago, Kurt and Terry traveled to Sacramento with a group of members from the AIDS Service Foundation [ASF,

California] to lobby for the HIV/AIDS budget. One of their constituents went to the office of the Congress and explained why continued funding was necessary. The people of the Congress were totally surprised because they'd been thinking all along that HIV/AIDS patients could take a pill and be done with the disease.

The truth is that HIV still infects and kills a lot of people, even in countries like the U.S.—confirmed by CDC, over fifty thousand Americans are newly diagnosed with HIV every year. The disease remains a killer. While Kurt Weston deals with the fear of dying from AIDS by confronting it, others deal with their fear by surrendering to it, or by choosing to "veg out and live as if they were retired," as the photographer puts it. It would be easy for him to do the same, to just give up on his fight; to receive his disability check and live off his life. But that kind of surrender has never been part of his genes, not even at times when he has found himself on the brink of depression.

In that sense, Kurt Weston has always been a warrior, yet never considered himself to be one. Rather, the photographer has always thought of himself as more of a passive person and, in many ways, an introvert. The positive energy necessary for his becoming a warrior has come in stages, through his diagnosis and during his "battle" with AIDS. He believes that people are not born warriors, but rather they choose to learn how to become warriors in order to battle whatever obstacles life throws in their paths. "I think that [when] you're affected by certain life situations, you have to endure, and then you have to react appropriately," Kurt Weston explains his warrior attitude towards life and AIDS.

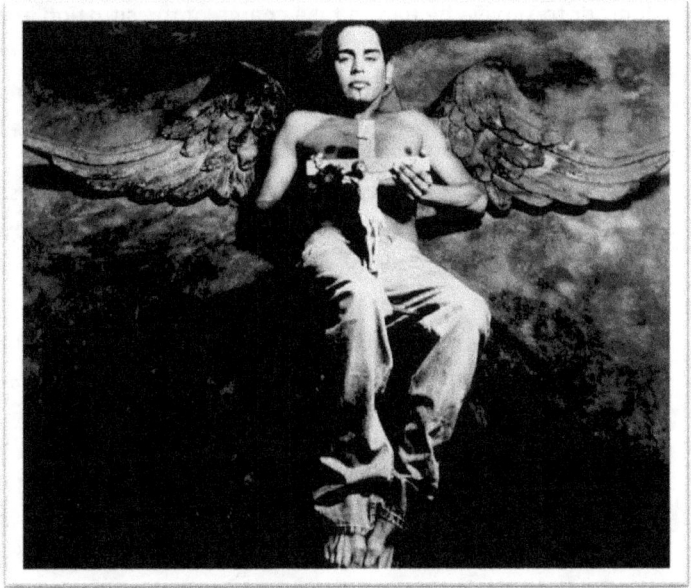

Prophet Angel

Some individuals just don't have it in their nature to respond in the way that's necessary for them to deal with a certain situation. And AIDS is not an easy situation to respond to, especially back when there were very few options and when an AIDS diagnosis wasn't a very promising scenario in terms of what the outcome would be.

Kurt Weston learned very quickly that he was either going to sink or swim, that he was either going to succumb to the disease or he could read everything he could find available about AIDS and realize that there was a lot that he could do to affect his future in a positive way. He learned that in order to survive he had to take charge of the situation and to believe that in some way he could affect the outcome of his AIDS. He also realized that he needed to be realistic and not live in denial when it came to his chances of staying alive.

Weston started his education in surviving his disease by looking at Buddhism and trying to understand how acupuncture, yoga, tai-chi or other experimental treatments and therapies could help him. He studied and absorbed as much information as he could regarding the benefits of taking herbs or vitamins, and he became familiar with the whole spiritual philosophy about Buddhism, yoga, and tai-chi.

In time, this abrupt learning process gave him hope and strength. Today, Weston believes that the alternative treatments really did help him. Trying them, despite the controversies surrounding their usefulness, has made him feel that he wasn't just waiting idle for AIDS to take his life, rather he was actively trying to do something proactive to ensure that he would continue to survive, that he did not limit his choices to the only existing conventional treatment, which was not very hopeful and had a lot of side effects. Besides, there weren't a lot of options in terms of taking only pharmaceutical therapy to start with.

To this day, the photographer believes in the importance of using complementary therapies, like vitamins and nutrients, in addition to the conventional drug treatments. Nutrients help strengthen the body. During an extended disease process, the body becomes incapable of assimilating nutrients properly, causing the wasting syndrome that used to be associated with HIV/AIDS; therefore, in order to reduce wasting, patients would need to take necessary nutrients in a concentrated form.

Yoga and acupuncture have also allowed Kurt to connect to his own body and learn to redirect more energy to the parts of his body that needed it most. This learning experience made him very conscious about his physical body and how it is connected to his inner, spiritual self. Today, the photographer believes that these realizations and experiences were vital for his surviving.

In time, with his health improving, Kurt found inspiration in helping others. Focusing on helping improving others' wellbeing gave a new sense to his existence. Throughout the years, he began to realize that he could help people and make a difference in many ways, through his Positively Speaking workshops, Very Special Arts or his artwork, which is inspired by his AIDS and vision loss. Trying to reach out to others, he realized that he could use all types of vehicles of communication to inspire or generate a dialogue with other people or make others aware of real life issues they might not have otherwise thought about.

Today, Kurt Weston hopes that his artwork benefits humanity, as effectively as both his speaking engagements and his continuing advocacy for helping people maintain a positive attitude towards life. "I think, by providing this type of service you start to forget about this selfish world, about what you need and what you want," Weston says. "It makes me feel very good and keeps me going when I see that people are thankful for things that I'm willing and able to do. I feel like I'm really accomplishing something."

The artist has taught himself the art of staying positive and hopeful by focusing on things in his life that he had wanted to achieve even before he got AIDS or become legally blind. Goals, like his art photography career, have kept him going and today he's thankful to have had this kind of inspiration in his life.

And although AIDS and legal blindness have made it even harder and more frustrating for him to achieve his goals, he has continued to focus on them. He has kept using his disabilities as sources of inspiration for his artwork through which he hopes to change people's perspectives on living with AIDS or with blindness and to show people that such disability subjects can be used as an art form. "Art is a big inspiration that keeps me going," Weston says, "I really thank God that I have this kind of inspiration in my life."

As a volunteer in the Positively Speaking HIV Prevention program in Orange County, Kurt Weston visits schools and talks to students about HIV/AIDS and, in particular, its impact on the young generation. The photographer always makes a point to advise students about the importance of following the career of their dreams, of their heart. He knows what can happen if they don't, if they only follow the money trail and end up in jobs they don't love, because it happened to him, too. He did not follow his career dreams from the very beginning and ended up doing a job he wasn't happy about. And so he started looking for happiness in all the wrong places—drugs, unsafe sex or other destructive behaviors.

"If you don't love your work, you'll look for love outside work and end up doing stupid things to feel good," Weston tells his students. "The chosen path in one's career has more to do with what you want to do with your life than one may think."

Today's students are faced with big decisions in their professional lives. They spend years studying and trying to figure out their future, and sometimes there is no crystal ball to tell them which direction to take in their career paths. The only compass they have available is their dreams, their hearts' desires.

Some students may have to try taking various courses to find out what they would love to do in life, while others may strictly follow the money trail, with no regards to what subjects actually interest them. All Kurt Weston can hope for is that people are able, eventually, to discover the paths leading to their lives' passion, like he did with visual art. His passion for photography allowed him to survive AIDS and blindness. Without this passion, he would have died a long time ago if he continued to work at Hartmax. For Kurt Weston, art is a motivation for living.

But other people may not be able to find the motivation or the strength necessary to survive something as extreme as a life-challenging disease, handicap, or calamity. While AIDS manifests differently in different people, patients also react in various ways to the disease and to the amounting obstacles that it throws in their lives.

Such is the story of a Los Angeles man, a story Weston heard on the radio... The man had had the disease for as long as Kurt had, and he had become resistant to all available medications... all but Fuzeon. But instead of starting self-administering his daily shots of medication, he decided to take a final and indefinite drug holiday and travel across the country in an RV with the decision to let the disease take over.

Meanwhile, a production company found out about him and decided to do a documentary on the patient's last days alive. So the video crew followed him as he started on his trip.

By the time he made it to New York, he started feeling sick and depleted of energy. So he had to purchase a plane ticket to return to L.A. He did, and once back on the West Coast he rented an apartment, and then committed suicide. The radio show played the last interview they had with him just before his suicide.

"I was completely disgusted," Weston comments. "Because I thought to myself, I've lived with [the same] disease for as long as this guy. I probably dealt with more than this guy did. I know that he wasn't possibly legally blind because he could drive himself across the country, which I can't do anymore. And yet, he didn't have the inspiration to continue his life."

What bothered the photographer even more was that the team of people recording the story thought that this person's decision to end his life was even worth a story to tell. To Weston, their action meant that profiling somebody who was giving up was more worthy than following the story of someone who was trying to do something positive and who was inspired to continue living.

Kurt Weston considers himself lucky that he has so much to live for. His life may not always be inspiring and joyful, but he is happy to still be able to pursue his goal, creating his art and achieving his dreams. This doesn't mean that he doesn't get depressed at times, but he also figured out a way to maintain a positive attitude towards life. Weston considers that thinking too much about oneself is a reason for depression. When that happens, he encourages people to think of those less fortunate, of the poor kids whose parents died from AIDS, of those living with famine and starvation and are dying from lack of water and lack of nutrition. Every time one thinks like that, it really is hard to even think of being depressed.

Although people can always find somebody in the world whose situation is far worse than theirs, stopping at this realization should not be an option. The next step is to be proactive in using their creative energy to do something efficient and useful to help those who have less. The experience keeps them away from getting down. Depression leads to destruction ("the D word"), which is just the opposite of creation ("the C word").

When he feels down, Weston starts thinking of being creative. He thinks about what he can do to add something to the world. For him, it really comes down to a "D and C" argument. For him, creation is the whole purpose of being an artist. And being an artist has kept him from thinking in destructive terms. Art has helped him survive his disease and his visual loss.

***

Nowadays, the artist is glad to find himself at a point in life where he feels that just surviving is not all he needs to be focusing on. But there were also times when it was vital for him to concentrate on his survival.

In the eighties and early nineties, some people didn't see it necessary to concentrate solely on their survival process. They thought that they could deal with the disease process while continuing their lives status quo. And they ended up dying because they didn't take the time to learn about their disease, to get in tune with all the parts of their inner universe and they did not take time to learn how to use their energy to get through the hurdle.

Some of Kurt's friends who had AIDS could never bring themselves to solely focus on their surviving. It cost some their lives.

Back in Chicago, Kurt had a friend, David, he hadn't seen in a long time. Kurt was already out on disability and starting his SWAN group at Test Positive Aware. Then, one day, David showed up at one of the meetings. Seeing his friend took Kurt completely by surprise. "When he walked in, I almost fell over because he looked absolutely horrible," the photographer recalls. "He had lost a tremendous amount of weight and he looked very, very ill. I could hardly recognize him."

Kurt knew that David had a company and that he was doing a lot of offset printing type of work for the Chicago Tribune. He fully expected David to tell him that he wasn't working anymore and that he'd sold his company and was trying to take care of himself.

"I'm still running my company," David said, instead.

"David, can't you see how bad you look and how sick you are?" Kurt asked. "Don't you think that people that you're doing business with can see how you look? Don't you think that they may think that you have AIDS or that there's something really terribly wrong with you?"

But David was in deep denial. He was convinced that he could continue being successful at his profession and also at staying alive. Determined to bring David back to reality and potentially save his life, Kurt took his friend to dinner and tried to talk to him and explain that he had to be more realistic about his disease, that maybe it was better to get rid of his company and start focusing solely on his health and his wellbeing. Yet, no matter how much Kurt would argue, David was unable to realize that he could, indeed, live without his job. Three or four weeks later, he ended up dying.

The news reminded Kurt how lucky he had been to realize that, in order to survive, he needed to stop doing all the other stuff that, at the time, he really thought he had to do… just like David had thought he had to do.

There were people Kurt knew who literally died on the job. Kurt's partner, Terry, knew someone at his work who was sick and who kept coming to work… until one day, when he didn't show up anymore. It turned out, he had died of AIDS and he had never admitted his disease to anybody.

Another one of Kurt's friends who was working and trying to survive his AIDS at the same time also died on the job. He had to go on a business trip and he got on the plane and died on the plane, while they were in the air.

These stories don't really happen anymore. HAART regimens have changed all that. Today, AIDS patients who've always taken the antiretroviral medications usually don't get so seriously sick anymore to be forced to stop everything else that's going on in their lives and concentrate solely on their survival.

Weston's AIDS diagnosis has reprioritized his life, reducing it to pure survival. His career took second priority, as did other aspects of his existence. What remained was his intrinsic desire to survive, which demanded his full and undivided attention.

It also required Weston to make a shift in consciousness, to realize that his life had to go into survival mode. It hasn't been easy to change his mindset, to actually realize the importance of switching priorities from the safety of a regular day job to the insecurities of living without a job and with a terminal disease. In the end, his survival instinct won and allowed him to let go of the life he knew and to go out on disability and, with that, into a life full of insecurities and unknowns.

Once he has begun nurturing his physical and spiritual being, he has also started tapping into all sorts of metaphysical philosophies that later influenced his artwork. After a while, his health became stable enough to allow him to resume his life from where he'd left off when AIDS had hit. Only first, he had to relearn how to live with his disease and, a few years later, with his visual loss.

Today, the artist talks about his hopes for the future, for his art and life. He believes that stem-cell research will be an integral part of finding a cure for AIDS, one that will come from some type of genetic therapy. Until then, he reminds, there is so much work to be done.

Kurt Weston also believes in the resurrection of a person's personal and professional life. Surviving and living with his AIDS represent only one part of the artist's own resurrection. By becoming a visual artist, he also resurrected his artistic career.

Weston's artwork, in particular his AIDS-inspired body of work, has a lot of iconic imagery and references to mythology. It is also rich in symbolisms. Inspired by the play Angels in America, Prophet Angel expresses the prophecy of AIDS epidemic. In the photograph, the angel is holding a crucifix, which symbolizes his modern crucifixion, because the person in the photograph is HIV positive himself. While angels are associated with the resurrection and ascension of the Christ, Weston's angel professes the resurrection of AIDS and, by extension, of any other terminal illness.

"I think that when you're living with a terminal illness you really are very conscious that the physical reality is not the only reality," the photographer comments. While finding himself so often on the brink of death, Weston became very conscious of the multi-dimensional reality—from physical to metaphysical—surrounding him. When he started to work with his chi, while at SWAN, he also learned that his life energy usually extends beyond the physical realm. Years later, this chi—his life energy—started to inspire his artwork.

Also, while making hospital visits to see people who were dying and who were also very spiritual—like the yoga teacher and tai-chi instructor—Kurt learned that they, too, were experiencing life on multiple dimensions. They were talking the language of people who understood life as a greater, more in-depth process, and perceived life on a deeper level. These people have influenced Kurt's life and artwork like his Blind Vision series of self-portraits, meant to be somehow abstract and quite figurative, thus adding a metaphysical dimension to his journey through darkness.

"I am sort of there but not really there," the photographer explains, talking about Blind Vision. "I'm kinda half in physical state and half in metaphysical state. Not completely solidified." The artist appears with his eyes closed, enveloped in blackness. The streaks running through the picture (the foam sprayed on the glass) simulate a stream of consciousness, portraying the artist's metaphysical journey through eternal blackness.

Nowadays, the artist continues using his life's experience to create art that is dynamic, informing, and also transforming. Weston believes that art has that kind of power, to make a difference in people's perception of life and its realities. "I want to continue making visual art that creates a consciousness shift when people look at it," he says.

Weston also believes that dreams, like art, are necessary in life, as is the struggle to make them true and see them become real. Sometimes, even more important than their dreams is the life journeys people need to take in order to reach their dreams. Also important is the transformational process they go through while on their journeys, even if they may not always be able to actually fulfill their dreams.

It's hard for anyone to predict the future, but Kurt Weston hopes for a bright one for his art and his life. Therefore, his dream is to continue to create art.

Sometimes, life's goals change and so do individuals' journeys through life. In that sense, Kurt Weston will always be searching for new ways of depicting his reality through his art and discovering new ways he has yet to explore. Kurt's art is always evolving because, as the artist comments, "it's not good for anybody to remain static." For Kurt Weston, creating visual art will always be an ongoing, life-long process. It will continue to expand and change and show itself in different ways. Ultimately, it will remain inspirational and transforming.

Appendix A: CMV Retinitis at a Glance

Flashing lights, floating spots, speckles of cotton before the eyes disturbing the sight, making it hazy and blurry as if you're looking through a screen may or may not be early signs of blindness. These symptoms may be the first signs of an eye disease called CMV retinitis.

Retinitis means infection of the retina, the thin layer of light sensitive tissue lining the back of the eyeball. The function of the retina is to convert the optical image we see with our eyes into electrical impulses that are further sent through the optical nerve to the brain. In the case of retinitis, even if the infection is cured, scars may remain on the retina. If left untreated, retinitis can lead to partial or total blindness.

Viral retinitis (caused by a virus) is most frequent in people with weakened immune systems, like HIV/AIDS patients or cancer patients (chemotherapy treatments can weaken immunity, making the patients prone to viral retinitis). There are three viruses that are commonly responsible for viral retinitis:

* Herpes simplex virus, which causes cold sores;

* Varicella zoster virus (HZV or Herpes Zoster Virus), which causes chicken pox;

* Cytomegalovirus retinitis, which causes total or partial blindness.

Cytomegalovirus is a kind of herpes virus that once inside the human body, it stays there for life. The virus is transmitted through bodily fluids like saliva, blood, urine, semen and breast milk, and lives peacefully in the healthy human body, in an inactive, (otherwise known as "dormant") state, not causing disease. Most people get exposed to CMV, especially with age, without being aware that they have been infected.

When the immune system weakens, CMV can become active. For example, in a person with AIDS, when the T cell count dips below fifty (a healthy individual has approximately one thousand T cells measured per unit of blood), CMV becomes active and can attack different parts of the body, causing serious damage. The virus can cause CMV retinitis in the eye or CMV pneumonia in the lungs and it can also spread to the esophagus, stomach, and bowels.

In AIDS patients, CMV most commonly affects the eye, causing CMV retinitis, an infection affecting the retina, which swallows and inflames. As a result, the signals sent from the eye to the brain become incomplete or inaccurate, leading to blurry vision or blind spots in the vision.

In some cases, people with CMV retinitis do not have any symptoms of the disease, sometimes even while they're on the verge of losing their sight. That's why it is advisable for people with very low T cell counts to go to an eye specialist for regular examinations and for a special test that checks for CMV in the eyes. Early lesions would look like small yellow-white patches with a grainy appearance, often accompanied by bleeding.

There are three standard medications used to treat CMV retinitis: ganciclovir, foscarnet, and cidofovir. CMV medications can be administered as intravenous (ganciclovir alone or in combination with foscarnet), intravitreal (injected into the vitreal fluid of the eye), as intraocular implants (surgically implanted into the eye to gradually release the drug), and also as oral medication. Oral medication is used for maintenance or as prophylaxis, to keep the CMV in check (inactive), thus reducing the risk of more damage to the retina and, therefore, preventing more vision loss.

HAART regimens, introduced in the mid-nineties, help keep the patients' immune systems healthy enough not to be prone to CMV infections. Therefore, with the advent of HAART regimens, the number of CMV retinitis cases among people living with AIDS has decreased by almost ninety percent.

Appendix B: Kurt Weston at a Glance

(Q&A Session with the Visual Artist)

Q. Who is your hero?

A. I have had many heroes throughout my life, but basically it is anyone who can take me to the next level of consciousness.

Q. What do you fear most?

A. Unrestrained hatred and prejudice.

Q. What/who inspires you?

A. Anyone who is inspired by reason, intellect, and compassion.

Q. What brings you hope?

A. Every hand that is extended towards mine, and every face that graces this world with a smile.

Q. What would you tell an aspiring artist?

A. Artists are creators; go create something that will transform people's perceptions.

Q. What are you most proud of?

A. Surviving AIDS and using my life experiences and my art to help others do the same.

Q. What is one of your bad habits?

A. I have an acute awareness of the passing of time and I become anxious unless I am using my time to continually do and create.

Q. Name one person/event/anything who's touched your life for the best? Worst?

A. This is a very complex question. I believe that there are different levels of consciousness that we experience over our lives and for each level there is a person who represents the best and the worst of humanity and life on this planet as we experience it. Currently my partner Terry is one of the best human beings I have ever had the pleasure of being connected with. And of course so many others before I reached this level with Terry. As for the worst, I believe that even what we consider as being terrible is placed in our path for a reason, even if the reason is to see the duality and polarity of the world we live in.

Q. What is the most useful thing you've learnt in life so far?

A. So much of our time is wasted on useless mind numbing activities, entertainment and trivial pursuits. The world belongs to people who are present, focused, and participating in life.

Q. Favorite (one) word to describe:

Art: Creation
Terry: Giving

Kurt: Being
Quasi: Unconditional
Va: Blossoming
Thomas: Intellect
SWAN: Surviving
TPA: Hope

Q. Favorite quote/motto you live by:

A. "And in the end the love you take is equal to the love you make." (John Lennon)

Q. Favorite word-phrase:

A. Wow!

Q. What do you want to be remembered by?

A. My artworks and fight to survive and thrive in the face of disease and adversity.

Q. What do you wish for in your life?

A. To use unrestricted resources to release the full potential of man's ability to cure disease, create transformative art, music and performance, and stop war.

Appendix C: "Warrior Within" originally

published in A&U Magazine--America's AIDS Magazine, November 2005 (the article that marked the beginning of our (photographer and writer) Journeys)

Warrior Within

By Alina Oswald

Photographer Kurt Weston works through AIDS-related visual loss to capture a portrait of the pandemic.

Photographer Kurt Weston sees his AIDS as a battle. And he needs to be a warrior willing to fight the virus that is destroying him.

"I never really wanted to just give up, even when I had the KS lesions. I think part of it was the fear of dying, but I didn't just wait for it to happen," he says, explaining his source of positive attitude during the course of our phone interview.

Diagnosed with full-blown AIDS in 1991, the award-winning visual artist considers protease inhibitors a miracle that literary saved his life. But, as he was restoring his health, he was also becoming legally blind, diagnosed with CMV retinitis in 1994.

"I was devastated because here I had spent my life working as a photographer and as a visual artist and I was no longer capable of doing this... or so I thought, because I couldn't see anything in focus. I don't see anybody's face," he says. "I see... like, if you look at the palm of your hand.

That's what I see of a person's face. So, I didn't think I could ever photograph again."

Fortunately, it turned out he could. And his first challenge was finishing the 1999 calendar for the Asian/Pacific Crossroads.

Many challenges later, after attending low vision technology studies at the California Braille Institute and experimenting with his new special equipment, Weston realized that he could, indeed, photograph. With the help of organizations like the Foundation for Junior Blind (now known as Junior Blind of America) and California Department of Rehabilitation, he purchased the special equipment— handheld telescope, special magnification glasses, and magnification and reading software programs like Zoomtext—necessary for him to continue his work.

"It was scary. A lot of times, I would take a leap of faith and do a lot of experimentation," he recalls this learning process.

Kurt Weston is a firm believer that a person can work through a situation, no matter how extremely challenging and helpless it may seem, and use the experience to help others who find themselves in similar circumstances. This philosophy has helped him work off the dilemmas in his own life while giving his life a deeper sense of meaning.

His early work in the AIDS community includes the founding of SWAN (Surviving With AIDS Network) a grass-root type of organization for people living with HIV/AIDS, as well as founding the Orange County Therapeutic Nutrients Program, which assists people living with HIV/AIDS.

One of the many ways Weston helps others today is through VSA arts (the Very Special Arts), an international organization committed to promote disabled artists. In June 2005, as a member of a VSA's Board of Directors, he went to D.C. with a VSA contingent to advocate for the continuation of funding because "this rigid administration and our wonderful President were trying to take all the money away from arts and education." He finds this absolutely appalling because these funds are vital for the careers of many potentially good artists.

From his perspective, Weston considers art a vehicle through which we can experience the nature of humanity. In today's society consumed by superficial realities, his art goes beyond the body and into a metaphysical dimension, connecting with the viewer on a more profound, spiritual level.

Kurt Weston's 2005 Unfinished Works award-winning work captures The Last Light of a dear friend. "He had AIDS and hepatitis," the artist explains. "He was seeing the light of day for the last time [because] two days after I took that picture he died. He had been a big light for many people and helped the HIV/AIDS community for many long years."

Peering through Darkness is part of Kurt Weston's Blind Vision series of self-portraits that show people the physical and emotional impact that visual loss can have on an individual. In order to represent his visual disturbance—

which he described like "pieces of cotton stuck in my eye, floating every time I move my eye"—he sprayed a glass with foaming glass cleaner and took a self-portrait sitting behind it. "You see my hand pushing away the foam, which is what I would love to do," he explains, "I would like to be able to wipe away all that cotton that keeps floating in front of my eye and get a clear view of what I want to see out in the world."

Weston believes that black-and-white offers his art a concentration of expression. And he likes that intensity, in particular in his portraits. He uses regular film and prints his images on silver gelatin paper so that they can last forever. He wants future generations to be able to look at this work and say, "This was happening at this time in history and this is the impact it left on people who's lives it touched, this pandemic."

But Kurt Weston is also concerned about today's young generation and the impact HIV/AIDS has on it. A volunteer in the Positively Speaking HIV Prevention program, he goes to schools and talks to students about HIV/AIDS.

"It's strange that people are ignorant about how they [might] get AIDS," he comments. "We need a lot more of [education and prevention]. Unfortunately, this [Bush W.] administration has fallen short in terms of discussing this issue. They basically only want people to know about abstinence. It would be nice if young people could abstain from sexual behavior, but that's not the reality. The reality is that a young person with hormones coursing through the body is going to engage in sexual behavior. And it's to [this kind of] individuals that we need to provide safer sex messages in terms of how to do it safely and prevent getting infected."

What about an AIDS cure? Kurt Weston believes that stem-cell research will be an integral part of finding a cure, one that will come from some type of genetic therapy. Until then, he reminds, there is so much work to be done.

NOTE: Find more of Kurt Weston's work by logging on to www.kurtweston.com.

Brief Glossary

ACT-UP: AIDS Coalition to Unleash Power, www.actupny.org

AIDS: Acquired Immune Deficiency Syndrome includes a complex of diseases determined by the deterioration of an individual's immune system.

Antiretroviral medications: ARV medications fight the virus by interfering with the growth and replication of HIV at various stages of its life cycle, thus prolonging the lives of those infected with HIV.

AZT: AZT (Azydothymidine) is the first mono-therapy antiviral drug, FDA approved in 1987

Bactrim: Bactrim is a wide-spectrum antibiotic and the most common medication used in treating PCP. It comes as an injection (IV) for acute cases of PCP and as tablets for maintenance and prevention treatments. One major side effect is that patients can become allergic to Bactrim and, therefore, forced to try other, sometimes less effective, PCP medications. Patients can be desensitized back to Bactrim, in pediatric (small) doses.

Cidofovir: This antiviral medication is similar to Ganciclovir in the way it works to keep CMV from multiplying. Cidofovir is available as intravenous injections (IV). One major drawback is its a negative effect on the kidneys. Usually, an infusion with a saline solution is necessary before the use of Cidofovir.

CMV: CMV, or cytomegalovirus, can enter an individual's body in a variety of ways, including by touching the eyes with unclean fingers. Once inside, CMV remains in the body for life, in an inactive, dormant state. When an individual's immune system starts deteriorating and its T-cell count deeps below a certain level (50), CMV can become active. CMV can infect different organs: the eyes, lungs, esophagus, or bowels. In AIDS patients CMV mostly attacks the eyes, causing CMV retinitis, which, if left untreated, can lead to partial or total blindness. Medications used for treatment of CMV retinitis include Ganciclovir, Foscarnet, and Cidofovir.

Entry Inhibitors: The role of entry inhibitor medications is to keep HIV from entering the T cell. One example of entry inhibitor is Fuzeon (T20), available only as an injection administered under the skin, usually twice a day. Other entry inhibitors include Maraviroc and Vicriviroc.

Foscarnet: This antiviral medication prevents CMV multiplication. It can be administered intravenously in a health care facility or at home.

Ganciclovir: This is one of the earliest and first medications used for CMV treatment. This antiviral drug helps to treat or prevent infections caused by CMV by keeping the virus from multiplying. Ganciclovir comes in three forms: intravenous, intraocular insert, and capsules. The capsule form is used for maintenance and prevention therapy only.

HAART: Highly Active Anti-Retroviral Therapy (or Treatment) regimens (a.k.a. HAART, pronounced like "heart" and sometimes referred to as ART—Anti-Retroviral Treatment) consist of a combination of three (or sometimes four) anti-HIV drugs. Also known as "the cocktail," HAART regimens have radically changed the progression of the disease. HAART regimens have the so-called "Lazarus effect" on AIDS patients, turning AIDS from a death sentence into a manageable, life-long disease. The new medications started being FDA approved in 1996. (Some mention December 7th, 1995, as the "discovery" date of HAART regimens.) Medical professionals need to constantly monitor their patients in order to make changes to their treatments to prevent patients from developing resistance to one or more drugs part of the specific drug regimen.

HIV: Human Immunodeficiency Virus is a human virus that causes the weakening of an individual's immune system by attaching itself to a protein on the T cell, called CD4. Once inside the T cell, HIV uses its own genetic material to make copies of itself. The T cell is destroyed in the process.

Immune System: The immune system's role is to keep the infections away from the body and/or to fight the infections already in the body. It achieves that through a complex array of organs, cells and molecules distributed throughout the body in places like the bone marrow, thymus gland, lymph nodes, spleen, and tonsils. T cells represent one type of cells whose function is to coordinate how the immune system fights infections.

Kaposi's sarcoma: KS is a tumor of the blood vessel walls. During the early years of the epidemic, it used to be the most common cancer in people living with AIDS. KS usually appears as pink, red or purple lesions on the skin, in the mouth or internal organs. KS can be treated with radiation and/or chemotherapy. Usually, lesions disappear once the immune system starts to recover (T cell count increases over a certain number).

Mepron (Atovaquone): Mepron comes in tablets or oral suspension. It is used to treat mild to moderately severe PCP in patients who are allergic to Bactrim (which is the standard therapy for PCP). Side effects include skin rash and fever. Most common ones are insomnia, diarrhea, cough, headache, and nausea or vomiting, also lack of energy, and fatigue.

NNRTIs: Non-Nucleoside Reverse Transcriptase Inhibitors (a.k.a. Non-NUKES) are medications that inhibit the reverse transcriptase enzyme by binding directly to the enzyme. NNRTIs include: nevirapine (Viramune) and efavirenz (Sustiva).

NRTIs: Nucleoside analogue Reverse Transcriptase Inhibitors (a.k.a. NUKES) represent the earliest antiretroviral drugs. They act by incorporating themselves into the DNA of the virus and blocking an enzyme called reverse transcriptase, which HIV needs in order to replicate. NRTIs include: zidovudine (Novo-AZT, Retrovir), lamivudine (Epivir, 3TC), and stavudine (d4T, Zerit).

PCP: Pneumocystis carinii pneumonia (most recent name is pneumonia jiroveci) is a lung infection commonly seen in people with compromised immune system. PCP, otherwise known as AIDS pneumonia, usually occurs in patients with a T cell count below 200. As in the case of CMV (cytomegalovirus), the organism that causes PCP can enter the healthy human body and live peacefully in it for the rest of its life, not causing any damages. Only when the immune system weakens or deteriorates, the organism activates and can cause pneumonia. In the early days of AIDS, PCP was too often a regular cause of AIDS related death for AIDS patients. Medications used for treatment of PCP include: Bactrim, Pentamidine, Mepron (Atovaquone), and Primaquine.

Pentamidine: It is used to prevent and treat PCP usually when the patient becomes allergic to the more commonly used antibiotic, Bactrim. Pentamidine is available in inhalation (for PCP prevention) and injection, or intravenous (for PCP treatment).

Protease Inhibitors: Protease Inhibitors, or PIs, inhibit replication of HIV protease, which is an enzyme needed for formation and assembly of HIV proteins. An example of PI is indinavir (Crixivan).

T cells: Also called CD4 or T helper cells, T cells are part of the immune system cells. Their role is to recognize—and then coordinate attacks against—any foreign invaders like bacteria, viruses, or fungi.

T cell count: T cell count [or sometimes T count] measures an individual's immune system. It is calculated per unit of blood. A healthy person's T cell count can vary but it's usually approximately one thousand (to twelve hundred). .

Viral Load (VL): Viral Load measures the amount of HIV in the patient's blood. Two tests—T cell count and Viral Load—

measure the evolution and the stage of the HIV infection in a patient's body. A low T cell count and a high viral load determine an advanced stage or progression of the disease. HAART regimens can keep the viral load at an undetectable level and the T cell count close to the normal range.

Acknowledgments

I attended my first AIDS conference in Eastern Europe as my mother's guest—she is a physician specializing in infectious diseases. It was April 1986 and I was on my spring break. At the time I felt pressured to decide what I wanted to do in life, but I wasn't planning to follow in my parents' footsteps and study medicine. By then all I knew about AIDS was the Rock Hudson story and his "before" and "after" AIDS diagnosis pictures splashed all over glossy magazines.

I remember sitting on the couch in my room, in my parents' apartment, flipping through the glossy pages of Paris Match (a French publication), opening it right in the middle. On the left page, a young and handsome Rock Hudson displayed the star-like smile everybody knew. The right page displayed the portrait of a gnawed-faced, almost unrecognizable actor—with his eyes ghostly, his appearance somber, like a much older version of the handsome actor on the opposite page.

What kind of disease could do this to a person, seemingly in no time at all?

That particular April afternoon I entered the building of the university of medicine—an old building with prestige, in an architectural style of its time, with a personality of its own—and sat next to my mother in a tall, dim-lit spacious room with no idea of what I was getting myself into.

"What do you think?" Mom asked several hours later, when the conference was over.

I looked at her and all I could say was, "Interesting."

I didn't know, then, that at the time I was attending the AIDS conference, a Los Angeles man was being diagnosed with AIDS and given only months to live. His name is Joel Rothschild and I was to meet him almost two decades later.

Several days after attending the AIDS conference, Chernobyl happened and plagued most of Europe, disturbing many people's lives in the worst possible ways. We found out about the explosion while listening to a radio station from Western Europe—I believe it was one of the Scandinavian countries that was first to announce the disaster. It all happened in the week before Orthodox Easter, when most people clean, cook, bake and work from dawn to sometimes dusk to get ready for the holiday.

In the middle of it all, water was turned off for several days. Fresh market products became unusable; therefore freshly bought milk, vegetables and fruits found their way into the trash containers. Picnic plans were canceled, although some individuals still went through with their already scheduled outdoor activities and enjoyed stretching on the irradiated grass.

TV and radio did not offer much information about the explosion, about what had really happened to those working at the nuclear plant or how many of them were dead or how we could stay safe. While at school, teaches would tell students to "lie flat on the street, by a sidewalk, and the wave of radiation [would] pass right above [your] body"! With the media forced to present the effects of the catastrophe as "nothing to worry about," many people had to learn more practical information through word of mouth and people who had some knowledge about the reality and implications of the disaster.

Shortly after the Chernobyl accident, oncology centers, especially those at the border with the (then) Soviet Union, filled with patients. Cancer survivors were getting sick again, especially children and the elderly.

Meanwhile scientists kept busy measuring the levels of radiation in the grass, in food, and people. Apparently in no time at all, every layperson became an "expert" in reading and interpreting the radiation tests. In addition, every individuals had their own version of the truth, insisting that theirs was the right one, the true story of whatever had happened at the Chernobyl plant.

Stories started to spread like a plague, while the few and selected individuals who knew the grim reality and its implications, and the toll we were to pay during the decades to come were forced to keep quiet, silenced by an administration of terror and oppression, by a government that would accept nothing else but pure perfection, utopia, even if it was all fakery.

In the midst of these events, the AIDS conference became kind of a blur. Little did I know then that the impact of that conference was going to follow me across an ocean and two continents, and guide me along both my professional—and personal—life.

My attending the 1986 AIDS conference wouldn't have been possible without my mother. So, thanks, Mom, for that opportunity and for everything else. Thank you and Dad for being the most wonderful parents and for helping me out with all medical terms for this book project. Most of them I can barely pronounce.

Thanks a million to my editor, Ira Weitz, for all your dedication and time you took to edit my manuscript, its every page, line, and word. Thanks for motivating me to finish "just one more" round of edits and, ultimately, this book project. Words are not enough to express how much I appreciate you believing in me, being the greatest "sillyologist" friend I've ever had. Thanks for always cheering me up, while trying to bring out the philosophical side of me.

Many thanks to Patricia Spork for being brave enough to publish my first essay so many years ago. To this day you're still keeping me on the write track. Thanks for your ongoing friendship, emails, phone calls, and encouragements. Also, thanks for your input and advice you so kindly offered while reviewing my drafts.

I also want to thank Joel Rothschild for being an inspiration and for giving new purpose to my life, in general, and my writing, in particular. Thanks to T.J. Banks for being there for me and for always being a wonderful friend.

Thanks to all of you who've read and reviewed various drafts of the book and offered opinions, ideas, and quotes. Much appreciated.

Last but definitely not least... Thank you, Kurt Weston. Journeys wouldn't have been possible without you. You took the time and patience to share your story with me. Thanks for being my inspiration and a great friend. I cherish every moment of the experience.

Alina Oswald, 2010

Notes on Sources

Interviews:

* Joel Rothschild, www.joelrothschild.com: August 2003

* Kurt Weston, www.kurtweston.com : September 2005; April 23, 2006; May 12, 2006; May 16, 2006; May 30, 2006; June 5, 2006; June 13, 2006, May 2007

* Interviews with cast members of RENT, November 2005

* Thomas Peterson, Director of Public Policy, AIDS Services Foundation, Orange County, www.ocasf.org , www.ocaidswalk.org, May 2007

* Infection disease specialist, Aurora Neacsu, MD and anesthesiologist Lucian Neacsu, MD, May-June, December 2006

* Interviews with psychologist Wolfgang Zaworka, Ph.D., Hamburg, Germany, October, December 2006

Workshops:

* Planning Council Meeting, Hudson County HIV/AIDS Office and Hyacinth AIDS Foundation, Jersey City, NJ:2006-2007

* HIV/AIDS Updates workshop at the LGBT Community Center, NYC: 2007

* HIV/AIDS Updates workshop for GMHC volunteers, GMHC, NYC: 2005

Books/Literature:

* The Johns Hopkins Complete Home Guide to Pills & Medicines

* Glossary of HIV/AIDS-Related Terms, Second Edition

* The Death and Afterlife Book—The Encyclopedia of Death, Near Death, and Life After Life, by James R. Lewis

* And the Band Played On, by Randy Shilts

* Hope—A Story of Hope, by Joel Rothschild

* Signals—An Inspiring Story of Life After Life, by Joel Rothschild

* Witness to AIDS, by Supreme Justice Edwin Cameron

* Angels in America, by Tom Kushner

* Freddie Mercury, by Peter Freestone

Films/Documentaries:

* Angels in America (HBO)

* And the Band Played On (HBO)

* The Age of AIDS (PBS)

* A Closer Look (PBS)

* RENT (Broadway musical, DVD)

Online HIV/AIDS Research Resources:

* The Body, www.thebody.com

* Visual AIDS, www.visualaids.org

* HIV Mirror, www.hivmirror.com (genetic test for disease progression)

* http://www.med.utah.edu

* www.hivinsite.org

* HIV Positive: www.hivpositive.com

* AIDS Map: www.aidsmap.com

* AIDS Education and Training Center (AETC): www.aids-ed.org

* Project Inform: www.projinf.org

* FDA: www.fda.gov

* CDC, Center of Disease Control: www.cdc.gov

* AIDS Treatment Data Network: http://www.atdn.org/simple/pcp.html

* John Hopkins Point of Care Center: www.hopkins-aids.edu

* On alternative treatments: www.yogavision.net, www.hps-online.com

Updates

In 2010 Terry and Kurt had to take Quasi to the vet for one last time. Quasi lived a long and good life.

Ambrose is a huge yellow lab and Kurt's guide dog. He came into Kurt's life in the summer of 2007.

Kurt graduated and now is teaching photography. A compilation of works from his Blind Vision series and Hearts of a Silent Age series is featured in Sight Unseen, an international art show (2009-2015).

In December 2011, Kurt and Terry (and Ambrose) visited New York City. Kurt was one of the top ten winners of Fight HIV Your Way photography contest and received a trip to Manhattan, to see the Alvin Ailey Dance Theater performance. I got a chance to see Kurt and Terry again, and meet Ambrose.

Kurt and Terry continue to make a difference in many people's lives

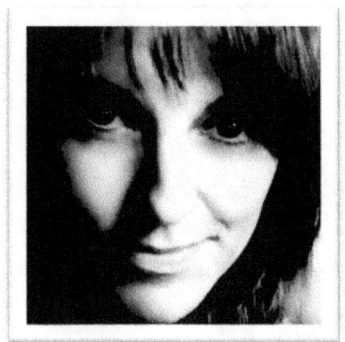

About the Author

Alina Oswald is a writer/photographer covering unconventional, inconvenient and sometimes taboo topics that populate human reality and imagination. Alina Oswald has documented the HIV/AIDS and LGBT communities for a decade, and her works have appeared in related publications and art shows. Her books include Vampire Fantasies, a collection of vampire-inspired photography, The Awakening…, a poetic photographic collection and Backbone, a collection of images celebrating unsung LGBT and HIV/AIDS heroes. Contact her online at www.alina-arts.com or follow her blog, Unconventional—Expressions of Reality, at alinaoswald.blogspot.com.

Contact Kurt Weston at www.kurtweston.com